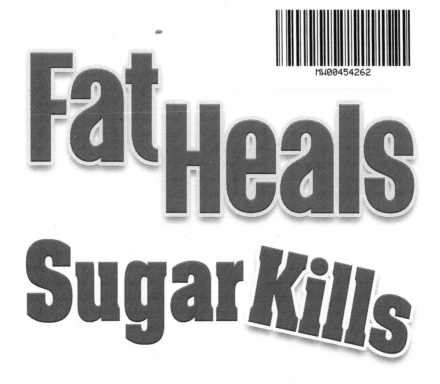

Fat Heals Sugar Kills

The Cause of and Cure for Cardiovascular Disease, Diabetes, Obesity, and Other Metabolic Disorders

By
Dr. Bruce Fife

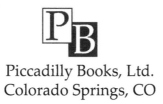

Piccadilly Books, Ltd.
Colorado Springs, CO

Piccadilly Books, Ltd.
P.O. Box 25203
Colorado Springs, CO 80936, USA
info@piccadillybooks.com
www.piccadillybooks.com

Library of Congress Cataloging-in-Publication Data

Names: Fife, Bruce, 1952- author.
Title: Fat heals, sugar kills : the cause of and cure for cardiovascular disease, diabetes, obesity, and other metabolic disorders / Bruce Fife, ND.
Description: Colorado Springs, CO : Piccadilly Books, Ltd., [2019] | Includes
    bibliographical references and index.
Identifiers: LCCN 2018056640 | ISBN 9781797654201 (pbk.)
Subjects: LCSH: Ketogenic diet. | Lipids in human nutrition. | Oils and fats,
    Edible--Health aspects. | Chronic diseases--Prevention.
Classification: LCC RM222.2 .F444 2019 | DDC 613.2/5--dc23 LC record available at https://lccn.loc.gov/2018056640

Contents

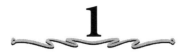

1

A Big Fat Mistake

BACK FROM THE GRAVE

At 390 pounds (177 kg) Reyn was a heart attack waiting to happen. In January 2015 he suffered heart failure and was admitted to the cardiac intensive care unit. After 12 days, he was discharged from the hospital with an oxygen tank. Although he lost a few pounds while he was in the hospital, he left with 44 pounds (20 kg) of excess fluid that had backed up into his abdominal cavity and lungs, a common consequence of heart failure, and thus the reason for the oxygen tank.

Reyn had struggled with type 2 diabetes for 15 years. His doctor had him taking a multitude of medications, including statins for his high cholesterol; Levemir (a synthetic form of insulin), NovoNorm, and metformin to control his blood sugar; and Victoza to help him lose weight. He followed his doctor's dietary recommendations by eating a low-fat diet with a modest amount of lean protein, avoided saturated fat, and centered his meals around grains, fruits, and low-fat dairy. As long as he took his medications regularly, he was free to indulge in desserts and sweets occasionally, especially if they were sweetened with artificial sweeteners. Despite the medications and following his doctor's dietary advice, his health steadily declined and every year he gained more weight. It was just his luck, he bemoaned, to be born with so many "genetic" health problems. His future looked grim.

The month following his release from the hospital, he attended a health conference that featured many internationally acclaimed speakers. To his amazement, he learned about a novel form of diabetes management using a low-carbohydrate, high-fat (LCHF) diet. After the convention he listened to additional speakers on the internet, extolling the virtues of the LCHF diet, in particular Jason Fung, MD, who had been one of the featured speakers at the conference.

The LCHF diet was completely contrary to everything Reyn had been told about diet and health. This peculiar diet strictly limits high-carb foods, such as grains, starchy vegetables, and most fruits. The calories that would otherwise come from these high-carbohydrate foods are supplied by fat, so fat consumption is significantly increased. Most of the fat is saturated, with limits on polyunsaturated vegetable oils. Fatty cuts of meat and full-fat dairy are preferred over low-fat versions. Such a diet would be viewed with disdain by most doctors and dietitians, but only because they have been taught to believe in the low-fat approach to dieting.

We have been following the low-fat way of eating now for the past 40 years, and where has it gotten us? Fatter and sicker! As a society we are fatter now than ever before. Obesity is at an all-time high, and degenerative conditions such as diabetes, Alzheimer's, arthritis, fibromyalgia, asthma, and COPD are at epidemic proportions. The low-fat approach to better health has been a miserable failure.

A growing body of research is showing that a LCHF diet can balance blood sugar, improve blood cholesterol levels, lower elevated blood pressure, melt off excess body fat, boost energy levels, balance hormones, strengthen the heart, and much more. All of these conditions have generally failed to improve much with the low-fat approach. While medications may help relieve symptoms associated with the above conditions, the LCHF diet can accomplish the same thing and allow patients to get off the drugs and lead healthier lives.

Convinced that a LCHF diet could help him, Reyn made a dramatic change to his diet, eating full-fat foods; forgoing fruit, sugar, and grains; and adding extra fat to his meals. He got about 75 percent of his daily calories from fat, 15 to 20 percent from protein, and about 5 percent from carbohydrate. Reyn began to wean himself off his insulin and cholesterol medications until he stopped taking them entirely.

Reyn told his cardiologist he did not want to renew his prescriptions for statins and insulin because he was improving using his new dietary approach. His cardiologist scoffed at him for seeking answers to his problems from the internet and following the advice of Dr. Google. Despite his doctor's criticism, Reyn continued with his newfound diet. After a year on the LCHF diet, Reyn lost 117 pounds (53 kg). He lost this weight easily, without experiencing the constant nagging hunger and lack of energy that he had experienced with the low-fat, calorie-restricted diets he had used before. In fact, he enjoyed full meals and ate until he was satisfied and had more energy than he had had for years. Weight loss was never so easy.

Reyn's blood sugar levels improved dramatically. A common measure of blood sugar is the A1C test, which gives a person's average blood sugar value over a three-month period. Reyn's reading before starting the LCHF diet was 9.1—extremely high. A reading of 6.5 or higher indicates diabetes. He was severely diabetic. Normal is between 4.0 and 5.6. Prediabetes ranges from 5.7 to 6.4. Reyn's reading after one year was 5.9—a substantial improvement and nearly into the normal range. Before starting the diet he suffered with peripheral neuropathy caused by his diabetes; the pain and numbness in his legs and feet associated with this condition vanished completely.

His total cholesterol dropped to 193 mg/dl (5 mmol/l), and his blood pressure fell to 115/72, both of which are considered ideal. No more cholesterol-lowering or blood pressure–lowering drugs for him! He essentially eliminated all of his medications with a simple dietary change that included full-flavored fatty meats, real butter, full-fat cheese, healthy oils, nuts, seeds, up to 20 eggs or more per week, and loads of vegetables covered in different full-fat sauces with a variety of herbs. A year ago, when he came out of the hospital, he literally had one foot in the grave. Today he feels great, is more physically active (swims 30 minutes a day, five times a week), is more cheerful, and has a positive outlook on life and on his future.

Reyn's story isn't an isolated incident; his success is being duplicated by many others who have regained their health with a low-carb, high-fat diet. You can have the same success.

LOW-FAT DIETS ARE KILLING US

In an effort to improve health and reduce the risk of heart disease, cancer, diabetes, and other conditions of growing concern, government health agencies set guidelines for their citizens on how to eat more healthfully. These guidelines state that we should eat more grains, vegetables, and fruits and less meat and fat. Grains, they say, should make up the bulk of our diet, consisting of 6 to 11 servings per day. This includes white and wheat breads, rolls, breakfast cereals, pancakes, muffins, crackers, cookies, oatmeal, rice, corn, cornbread, tortillas/chips, and like products. In addition, they say we should eat 3 to 5 servings of vegetables and 2 to 3 servings of fruit a day. Fried potatoes, pizza sauce, and catsup all fulfill the vegetable requirement. Sugary fruit juice, cherry pie filling, and canned fruits with syrup all satisfy the fruit requirement. We are told that milk and cheese should be limited to no more than 2 to 3 servings daily, and that we should stick with the nonfat or low-fat versions. Meat, fish, eggs, and nuts, likewise, should be limited to 2 to 3 servings, with emphasis on lean cuts of meat and preferably egg whites over whole eggs. Fats and sugar should be restricted to only "occasional" use, with saturated fat being all but eliminated from this scientifically approved "healthy" diet.

Dutifully we put forth our best efforts to follow this advice and have generally been successful. Since the 1970s we, on average, have increased our fruit and vegetable intake by 17 percent and our grains by 29 percent, and reduced the amount of fat we eat from 40 percent to 33 percent of calories, mostly by cutting out saturated fats. During this time we have also been exercising more—all according to recommendations given us from our doctors and government health agencies.

We are eating more reduced-fat, low-fat, and nonfat foods of all types, including lean cuts of meat, and using far less oil in cooking and food preparation. This reduction in fat has led to an increase in carbohydrate consumption because removing fat from meals generally leads to eating more carbohydrate-rich foods to make up for the loss of calories from fat. This means eating more wheat, rice, corn, pasta, potatoes, fruit, and juices. A typical breakfast of eggs and bacon has been replaced by sugary breakfast cereals and orange juice or pancakes with syrup and low-fat milk. White flour is our most commonly consumed carbohydrate; we eat it in a variety of ways, as bread or rolls, but more commonly as donuts, cinnamon rolls, cupcakes, pie crust, and all manner of sweets and desserts. The recommendation to reduce fat consumption and increase grain intake has consequently led to an increase in sugar consumption. Although the guidelines suggest limiting sugar intake, this advice is not stressed and has generally been ignored, with more emphasis placed on reducing total fat intake and cutting out saturated fat and cholesterol as much as possible.

The reduction of total fat has been accomplished primarily by giving up animal fats and tropical oils, both sources of saturated fat. This has led to the replacement of saturated fats with polyunsaturated vegetable oils. Consequently, vegetable oil consumption has significantly increased at the expense of saturated fats. Included among the vegetable oils are hydrogenated vegetable oils, shortenings, and margarine.

In an effort to cut down on saturated fat, cattle have been bred to have less fat so that they produce leaner cuts of meat. The meat you purchase in the store today is much leaner than the meat your grandparents bought back in the 1960s and earlier.

The low-fat, low-cholesterol diet was first officially recommended to the public by the American Heart Association in 1961. The diet was further refined over the ensuing years, culminating in the United States Department of Agriculture's Food Guide Pyramid, established in the early 1990s. Despite making all the recommended dietary changes over the years, our health has not improved. In fact, we are less healthy today than ever before. In the 1960s heart disease was by far the most common cause of death. One of the major goals of the low-fat diet was to reduce the risk of heart disease, yet 60 years later, heart disease is still our number one killer.

Stroke is the second leading cause of death worldwide, behind heart disease, and the fifth leading cause of death in the United States. High blood pressure (hypertension), a major cause of stroke, affects 1 in 3 American adults. The incidence of high blood pressure has steadily risen since the 1960s. In a single ten-year period, from 2000 to 2010, the number of deaths from high blood pressure rose 41.5 percent.

One of the major reasons given for the low-fat diet is to prevent obesity and to achieve better control over managing weight. However, it hasn't worked. In the 1960s only 1 in 7 American adults were obese. Today, that number has risen to 1 in 3. More than 70 percent of American adults are now overweight—the largest percentage in history. Even our children have gotten fatter: one-third are overweight and 17 percent are obese. Our growing obesity problem has become a national health crisis.

One of the most pervasive plagues of our day is diabetes. In 1960 fewer than 1 percent of American adults had diabetes; today that number has risen to more than 10 percent. The rate is even higher among seniors ages 65 and older, affecting 1 out of every 4. Additionally, 1 in 3 adults have prediabetes, as do more than 50 percent of those aged 65 or older. An estimated 80 percent of American adults have some degree of insulin resistance, the underlying

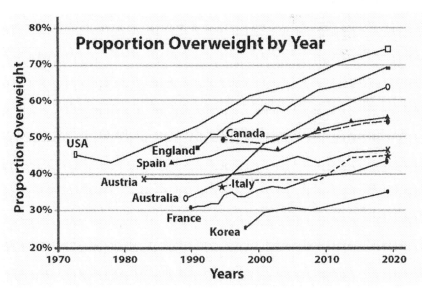

Overweight has become a worldwide epidemic.

9

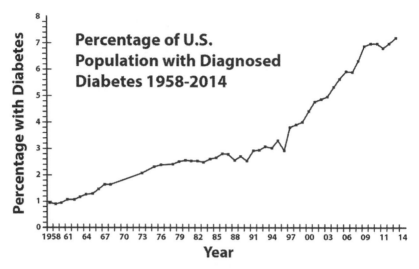

feature of type 2 diabetes. If current trends continue, researchers estimate that 1 in 3 Americans born in 2000 will develop diabetes in their lifetime. Diabetes is currently the seventh leading cause of death in the United States.

Diabetes rates in the United States were fairly stable, with only a slight increase from 1958 to 1962. Then suddenly, rates began a sharp upward climb, with another sharp upward shift beginning in the mid-1990s.

Type 1 diabetes is an inherited condition that makes up less than 10 percent of all diabetes cases. Type 2 diabetes is by far the most common form, accounting for at least 90 percent of cases. This type of diabetes is caused predominantly by a high-sugar, high-carb diet and sedentary lifestyle. In recent years, it has been discovered that Alzheimer's disease is another form of diabetes—diabetes of the brain. It is now referred to as type 3 diabetes. It, too, is caused predominantly by diet and lifestyle choices.

Currently, 1 in 6 women and 1 in 10 men who reach the age of 55 will eventually develop Alzheimer's. In just five years, from 2000 to 2005, the incidence of Alzheimer's disease increased by 44.7 percent. In 1991 Alzheimer's disease was recorded as the underlying cause of 14,112 deaths. By 2000 this number had increased to 49,558; by 2005 it had grown to 71,696, and by 2016 it was estimated that 700,000 people died from the disease.[1] A generation ago, death from Alzheimer's was less than 1 percent and wasn't even among the top 20 causes of death. Today it is the sixth leading cause of death in the United States.

It is not just diseases that lead to death that are increasing, but those that cause disability too. Glaucoma, macular degeneration, arthritis, fibromyalgia, multiple sclerosis, ulcerative colitis, celiac disease, infertility, and others are all on the rise. These conditions have been increasing rapidly over the past several decades, and rates continue to climb, thus ruling out a genetic cause. Genetic diseases don't suddenly appear out of nowhere and take over a population like a plague. While most of these conditions have probably existed to some extent throughout human history, up until recently they have been relatively rare.

Some claim that because of modern drugs and medical technology, people are living longer nowadays, and therefore, as the population ages, we are developing more old-age diseases than they had in the past. Unfortunately, these so-called old-age diseases are not restricted to the elderly. People are dying from heart attacks in their 40s and 50s, and some even earlier.

Type 2 diabetes used to be called *adult-onset diabetes* because it was only seen in older adults. However, over the years, younger and younger people have been diagnosed with diabetes, which is why the name was changed to type 2 diabetes.

Alzheimer's, too, was once considered strictly a disease of the elderly, but people in their 40s and 50s are now developing it. They call this *early-onset Alzheimer's*. In some cases it affects people in their 30s and younger. It seems that the disease can occur at nearly any age.

Not only are degenerative diseases on the rise, but so are childhood disorders, such as allergies, asthma, developmental disabilities, autism, childhood obesity, narrowing of the dental arch, and so on. These are clearly not consequences of an aging population.

So, what's happening here? We've been following the government's dietary guidelines for the past five decades, and as a result we have grown fatter and sicker. Conditions that were once rare or unheard-of a few decades ago are now commonplace. Obviously, something is terribly wrong.

The cause of this epidemic is not because we all overeat or we don't care about our health. The problem is that we have been given faulty advice about diet and health. The low-fat, high-carb diet so strongly promoted for the past several decades has been a disaster and has created a health crisis.

If you want to lose excess weight as well as reduce your risk of stroke, heart disease, atherosclerosis, cancer, and many other degenerative diseases, you should eat more fat and less sugar and refined carbohydrates. In fact, eating more fat may be one of the healthiest decisions you can make—if it is the right kind. Sound far-fetched? It's not.

We have been told that fat and cholesterol are the cause of ill health for so long that we have become thoroughly brainwashed into believing it. We need to stop thinking of fat as the enemy and make a complete paradigm shift in thinking about diet and health.

We need to consider the possibility that instead of being a villain, fat may be good for us and sugar might be the real troublemaker. Could this be possible? How could we know? History provides us with a clue.

Throughout history fat was an important and even essential component of our ancestral diet. Fat was savored, and every morsel of fat on game was harvested and eaten with relish. Sugar, on the other hand, was completely absent, or rarely eaten. People enjoyed excellent health and physical development on high-fat diets. However, during the 20th century, as fat consumption declined and sugar consumption increased, our health has suffered.

WHAT A LCHF DIET CAN DO FOR YOU

If you are worried about developing chronic degenerative disease as you grow older or if you already are experiencing symptoms of premature degeneration, a LCHF diet may be the solution you are seeking. Most chronic degenerative disease is caused or exacerbated by poor dietary choices. Unfortunately, the dietary advice we have been given for the past several decades has been a big fat mistake and has led us in the wrong direction.

Recent cutting-edge research is now showing that a low-carb, high-fat diet can reverse many of the adverse health effects caused by the low-carb diet. Some of the many conditions that can be stopped or reversed with a LCHF diet include:

allergic rhinitis	hypogonadism
Alzheimer's disease	infertility
asthma	insomnia
atherosclerosis	insulin resistance
cancer	kidney disease
cataracts	kidney stones
chronic fatigue	lupus
COPD	macular degeneration
coronary heart disease	metabolic syndrome
Crohn's disease	nonalcoholic fatty liver disease
depression	obesity
diabetes	osteoarthritis
epilepsy	Parkinson's disease
fibromyalgia	peptic ulcers
gallbladder disease	polycystic ovary syndrome
glaucoma	psychological disorders
hepatic steatosis	sleep apnea
hyperandrogenism	thyroid dysfunction
hypertension	ulcerative colitis
hyperuricemia	vascular dementia

The number and variety of conditions that can be benefited by a LCHF diet are incredible; this list doesn't include them all, but even so it represents the most frequently uncounted health problems of modern society. If you suffer from any of these conditions, a LCHF diet may bring about a remarkable change in your life. You will be able to get off most if not all of your medications, have more energy, be more resistant to infections, feel better, sleep better, have a clearer mind and a better memory, and experience an overall enhanced feeling of well-being.

A properly designed LCHF diet can be like hitting the reset button on your health. Years of poor dietary and lifestyle choices can be wiped away or greatly reduced, providing you with a fresh start on life.

The key here is a "properly designed" LCHF diet. Just adding more fat into your diet will not work. You must also reduce your carbohydrate intake, especially sugar and refined grains. The type of fat you eat is also important. Not all fats are of equal value, and some can be harmful, or harmful if eaten in excess. The proper amounts and percentages of fat, carbohydrate, and protein are also important, as is the source of these nutrients. This book will guide you through it all.

While it may look like a LCHF diet can correct just about anything, it is not a cure-all, nor do I claim it to be such. The diet itself doesn't cure anything; it simply provides the body with the nutrients it needs to correct imbalances caused by poor dietary and lifestyle choices. If you have been eating the standard low-fat diet, this new way of eating has the potential to significantly improve your health. It may just be the solution you are looking for. Give it a try—you have nothing to lose except your poor health.

2

Modern Diets and Degenerative Disease

A BIG FAT LIE

The warning to reduce consumption of fat, specifically saturated fat and cholesterol, is found everywhere we look. Doctors advocate very low-fat diets to help fight heart disease and other degenerative conditions. Over the past few decades, fat has emerged as the biggest threat to health that mankind has ever faced. Everybody blames their health problems on excess fat. It has become a convenient excuse. But how bad is it really? After all, people have been eating saturated fat and cholesterol for thousands of years. Why, suddenly, is it now considered a health problem when it wasn't before? Much of what we hear is nothing more than a big fat lie. Fat is actually a necessary part of our diet and a vital component of our bodies.

We often think that the less fat we have on our bodies and the less we eat, the better. If you weigh 150 pounds (68 kg), but are not overweight, your body would contain 30 pounds (14 kg) of fat. This fat serves an important purpose. We need it to be healthy. In fact, without it we would be dead. Fat provides a protective cushion for delicate organs, helps regulate body temperature by insulating us against environmental extremes, is involved in the production of vital hormones, and provides a readily accessible source of energy when food is restricted or physical activity is increased. Vitamins A, D, E, and K, as well as beta-carotene, lycopene, lutein, CoQ10, and other nutrients essential to good health and the maintenance of life, are only found in the lipid (fat) component of vegetable and animal foods. Fats, or lipids form a major part of the structure in all of our cells, particularly the cell membrane.

Every cell in our bodies must have a continual source of energy to keep it functional and living. This need for energy is so vital to the life of the cell that interruption even for a few minutes would bring death. This need for a continual supply of energy is satisfied primarily by the fat stored in our bodies. Fat provides the calories we need between meals and during times of prolonged fasting. Stored fat supplies about 60 percent of the body's ongoing energy needs when we are at rest. When exercising or during prolonged periods without food, fat stores make an even greater contribution to our energy needs.

One of the most important lipids in our bodies is cholesterol—yes, cholesterol, the so-called evil villain of the dinner plate. Cholesterol is so important to the basic operations of life that without it, every cell in the body would be dead. Cholesterol is found in all body tissues and comprises a vital part of the cell membrane. Nine-tenths of all the body's cholesterol is located in the external and internal membranes of cells. It is essential in the production of nerve tissues. It is used by the body to make bile acids necessary for digestion of fats and fat-soluble vitamins. We get most of our vitamin D from cholesterol. Our bodies transform cholesterol into a variety of important hormones, such as estrogen, progesterone, testosterone, DHEA, cortisol, and others. If we had no cholesterol, we would be sexless. That is, there would be no male or female differentiation, and reproduction would be impossible.

Cholesterol deficiency, however, is usually not a problem. Its presence is so vital to health that if we don't get it in our diet, the body will synthesize it in the liver from other nutrients. Your liver is manufacturing cholesterol right now at the rate of about 50 quadrillion molecules per second. The raw materials that the liver uses to make cholesterol can be derived from carbohydrate, protein, or fat (both saturated and unsaturated).

The body tries to maintain a balance between the amount we eat and the amount manufactured in the liver. If we eat little, then the liver will produce more. If we eat more, the liver produces less. This is why even drastic decreases in dietary cholesterol intake often produce only small drops in blood cholesterol levels.[1] If we eat too much, the excess is then broken down by the liver and converted into triglycerides (fat molecules) to be stored as body fat.

Fat is not the villain it is often made out to be; however, not all fats are alike. Some dietary fats are good for us, some are not so good, and others are downright dangerous. The problem is that many of the good fats are condemned as bad and the truly bad ones are praised as good. Even many health professionals are confused and lead people astray with erroneous dietary advice. Many people right now are consuming oils they think are good for them or at least not harmful, but are damaging their health.

THE FOOD REVOLUTION

Our ancestors subsisted on diets of fresh natural foods they made, killed, gathered, or grew. As long as they could get enough to eat, including good quality fat, they enjoyed relatively good nutritional health. Before the 1900s, people lived on fresh, whole foods that were grown or raised on local farms. As they moved from the farms into cities, the need to feed a growing population led to the development of mass production techniques. Foods were bottled, canned, and packaged so they would have a long shelf life, would last throughout the winter, and could be shipped long distances. As a consequence, foods became less nutritious and contained questionable additives.

Although nutritional deficiencies occurred from time to time, the most prevalent diseases were those caused by infectious microorganisms. Pneumonia and tuberculosis were the dreaded diseases of the day. Degenerative disease was comparatively rare. Most of the degenerative diseases that are common today were so rare that they were not even recognized at that time.

Louis Pasteur (1822-1895) ushered in a new era in science and preventative medicine with the discovery of germs—microscopic organisms that can cause disease. The cause of infectious illnesses that had plagued mankind from the beginning of time was at last discovered. The attention to sanitation and hygiene put a stop to many diseases that had plagued the world. In hospitals, the simple act of washing hands saved the lives of thousands of patients. Before that time, it was common for doctors when treating new patients to simply wipe their hands off on a towel after attending to a sick patient or even after dissecting a cadaver. As you might expect, people would come into a hospital for one condition and often die of another.

At the same time, a revolution in food technology began to take place. Food processing enhanced taste and prolonged shelf life. Rice was polished to remove the brown, fibrous outer layer. Wheat milling methods were developed that allowed a more thorough separation of fiber for a more refined, whiter flour. Sugar production became more cost-efficient, and production rates soared.

The dietary habits of the population began to change from one based on the whole, natural foods of our ancestors to one based on the highly processed foods of today. In 1800 we consumed about 15 pounds (72 kg) of sugar per person each year; by 1900 that amount had increased to 85 pounds (38 kg); by 1999 it had increased to more than 150 pounds (68 kg); today it has declined to about 130 pounds (60 kg), but only because of the increased use of artificial sweeteners and the growing popularity of low-carb diets.

Cold breakfast cereals, some of our first convenience foods, made their appearance in the 1890s, along with soda pop, ice cream, and other junk foods. By the 1970s the traditional breakfast of bacon, eggs, butter, and whole milk took a backseat to highly sweetened cereals, pancakes and syrup, pastries, low-fat milk, chocolate milk, and sweetened juices.

The fats and oils consumed by our great-grandparents were much different from those we typically eat today. Our ancestors ate butter, lard, or beef tallow along with some imported coconut and olive oils. Most of these fats were highly saturated. Vegetable oils, such as corn, soybean, safflower, and cottonseed, were rarely eaten before 1900 because of the expense involved in their production and their tendency to go rancid quickly. With the development of the hydraulic oil press, vegetable oils became more cost-effective and cheaper than the animal fats. In 1911 the invention of the process of hydrogenation led to the introduction of Crisco shortening and later margarine (both hydrogenated vegetable oils that contain harmful trans fatty acids). Shortening and margarine were touted as cheaper and "healthier" alternatives to animal fats. During the Great Depression of the 1930s these cheaper hydrogenated vegetable oils became widely popular as substitutes for the more expensive animal fats. Vegetable oil production steadily increased after World War II. By 1958 world vegetable oil production exceeded 60 billion pounds yearly.

Foods were processed and packaged to look appetizing, to tantalize the taste buds, and to have as long a shelf life as possible. In the process, nutrients were destroyed and natural and synthetic chemicals were added. You go to the store now and it's near impossible to find a packaged food that doesn't have sugar or sweeteners, preservatives, dyes, emulsifiers, anticaking agents, flavor enhancers, or other additives.

We learned as early as the late 1800s, after the practice of polishing of rice became common, that food processing can cause deficiency disease. This didn't stop the practice; we just added back some of the vitamins that were removed. This was a quick fix, but not a good solution. Some 22 nutrients are removed in the processing of wheat into white flour. Only four or five are added back. Scientists have now identified as many as 90 nutrients that are important to health. Modern food processing methods remove most of them.

In his book *Nutrigenetics*, Dr. R.O. Brennan lists how much of each nutrient is lost when whole wheat is converted into white flour; for example: magnesium (85 percent), provitamin A (90 percent), vitamin B_1 (77 percent), vitamin B_2 (80 percent), vitamin B_3 (81 percent), vitamin B_6 (72 percent), folic acid (67 percent), calcium (60 percent), vitamin E (86 percent), zinc (78 percent), and selenium (16 percent).[2] If you are like most people, you eat bread or flour of one type or another at every meal. This could be pancakes, tortillas, breakfast cereal, donuts, bagels, noodles, and so on. You might be surprised at how many flour products you eat every day. Wheat comprises the bulk of most of our foods. These products are almost always made from white flour.

Processed vegetable oils, sugar, and white-flour products make up 73 percent of the average American diet and supply almost no vitamins or minerals. When animals are placed on diets of refined and processed foods, they develop a long list of degenerative conditions, which increase in number and severity in successive generations. The relationships are so strong that specific nutrient deficiencies frequently can be shown to cause defects in specific parts of the body.[3]

The infectious diseases that plagued mankind in ages past have been controlled for the most part by antibiotics and improved sanitation. But a whole new breed of illness has taken their place. Degenerative diseases are now on the rampage. Diseases that were rarely seen before throughout all of human history have now become commonplace.

TRADITIONAL DIETS

The transformation of the major cause of death and disability from infectious disease to degenerative disease began in the early 1900s with the advent of the industrial food revolution. The rates of degenerative disease further accelerated beginning in the 1960s with the demonization of saturated fat and cholesterol and the adoption of the low-fat diet as our health standard.

If you go to areas of the world where people still eat traditional foods that they produce themselves, void of commercial processed products, you will find that these populations have a dramatically lower incidence of all types of degenerative disease. Heart disease, cancer, and diabetes are unknown to them—or were until recently. Now, however, as modern processed foods have been introduced into these populations, degenerative disease has followed. This pattern has been repeated time and time again throughout the world. As soon as a population starts to adopt modern foods, degenerative disease creeps in.

Degenerative diseases, such as heart disease, cancer, Alzheimer's, asthma, bronchitis, diabetes, arthritis, allergies, obesity, and the like, are referred to as "diseases of modern civilization." These conditions are rare among primitive societies who live on traditional diets consisting of whole, natural foods. When populations are introduced to modern civilization and adopt Western foods, diseases of modern civilization soon develop. Researchers and historians have found that within just a single generation these cultures experienced all of these degenerative conditions, clearly indicating that they are not caused by genetic defects.

The link between diet and the rise of degenerative disease was aptly demonstrated back in the 1930s by Weston A. Price, DDS (1870-1948). Dr.

Price served as the chairman of the research section of the American Dental Association from 1914 to 1923 and is noted for his extensive research on nutrition and dental health.

During his long career as a practicing dentist, Price observed an increasing incidence of tooth decay and dental deformities and other health problems late in his career that were rare in his earlier years. He was seeing more and more children with narrow dental arches and crowded teeth. When the wisdom teeth erupted, there often wasn't room for them, which required that they be extracted. This was a curious phenomenon because early in his career patients rarely had to have wisdom teeth removed. Remains of ancient humans show broad dental arches and healthy wisdom teeth. It didn't make sense that the human body, as perfectly designed as it was, would suddenly grow teeth that didn't work and required surgical removal. At no time in human history had there been a need to remove wisdom teeth from so many people. It wasn't just the teeth, he also noticed that the general health of his patients was declining; they were developing degenerative diseases at an increasing rate. He was seeing the so-called diseases of "old age" in younger and younger patients.

Price was a firsthand witness to the transformation and revolution of modern food processing. He wondered if the changes in the diet were related to the decline in health. He set out to find the answer. He began a series of studies comparing the health of people who ate traditional diets with those who ate modern, processed foods. To avoid other influences that may affect health, the people studied would be of the same genetic background and live in the same geographic area. The only difference would be the diet.

Today it is nearly impossible to find populations that rely solely on traditional foods. Modern foods are found virtually everywhere throughout the world. But in the 1930s there were still many populations that subsisted primarily on their ancestral foods, without modern influences.

Dr. Price spent nearly a decade traveling around the world, locating and studying these populations. He traveled to isolated valleys in the Swiss Alps, and the Outer and Inner Hebrides off the coast of Scotland. He visited Inuit villages in Alaska, American Indians in central and northern Canada, the Melanesians and Polynesians on numerous islands throughout the South Pacific, and tribes in eastern and central Africa. He also spent time among the Aborigines of Australia, Malay tribes on islands north of Australia, the Maori of New Zealand, and indigenous peoples of South America in Peru and the Amazon Basin.

When Dr. Price visited an area, he would examine the people's health, particularly their teeth. He made careful note of the foods they ate and meticulously analyzed the nutritional content of their diet. Samples of the foods were sent to his laboratory, where detailed analyses were made. It didn't take long for him to notice the contrast in health between those who lived entirely on indigenous foods and those who had incorporated Western foods into their diets.

Price found that the more isolated a native population was, the less tooth decay and other degenerative disease he found. In areas that were almost totally isolated, the natives had almost no tooth decay and the people were healthy and strong. Degenerative disease was virtually unknown to them. In areas that were easily accessible and Western influence was greater, tooth decay and disease were much more prevalent.

Price soon noticed a pattern developing. Tooth decay became particularly common among children in areas where modern processed foods were available. Price found that wherever white flour, white rice, and sugary foods were sold, tooth decay and degenerative disease were prevalent. He got to the point where he could tell how many years the local store had been in operation by the age of the children with the most tooth decay. He would go into a new area and, after examining the teeth of the children and comparing their ages, he could tell the year in which their store had opened.

Wherever Price found people living on traditional foods, he noted that both their dental and physical health were excellent, but when the people began eating modern, processed foods, their health quickly deteriorated. In the absence of modern medical care, physical degeneration was pronounced. Dental diseases, as well as infectious and degenerative diseases, such as arthritis and tuberculosis, were common among those eating Western foods.

The Western diet affected not only those who ate it, but also their unborn children. Parents who added modern foods into their own diet gave birth to children whose teeth and bone structure were improperly developed. Children were born with narrowed dental arches; when their teeth came in, they were crowded and crooked, and wisdom teeth became impacted. In contrast, those children whose parents ate traditional foods had excellent dental health and development. They possessed wide dental arches, had straight, healthy teeth, and wisdom teeth came in without problem.

The degeneration in health that was occurring in these primitive societies when they adopted commercially processed foods was the same that Price had been seeing in his dental practice. The connection was obvious. Modern, processed foods were nutritionally deficient, and consequently, people were developing a greater number of degenerative conditions and children were being born with developmental deficiencies.

One of Price's most frightening discoveries was that it didn't take much of a change in the people's diets to cause notable changes in health. While their diet remained primarily the same as it had always been, the addition of even a small quantity of sugar and white flour made dramatic differences in their health.

Another thing Price discovered was that the types of foods eaten varied greatly from one population to the next. Inuit and Canadian Indians ate a diet that consisted almost entirely of meat and fat. The Pacific Islanders consumed large quantities of fish, fruit, root vegetables, and fat (primarily from coconuts). The inhabitants of the islands off the coast of Scotland subsisted largely on oats and seafood. Those in the Swiss Alps relied primarily on dairy and unlike many other populations, never touched fish. Despite the wide variety in their diets, the one thing they did have in common was that the foods were fresh or fermented and relatively whole and minimally processed. There was no refined sugar or white flour. All fats were natural, consisting predominantly of saturated fats derived from meat, dairy, or coconut. There were no polyunsaturated vegetable oils used. The small quantity of honey or sugarcane a few populations may have eaten was seasonal and constituted only a very minor part of their overall diet.

The amount of fat in the diets of the people Price studied varied greatly. However, those who consumed the most fat and the least carbohydrate also had the least amount of dental decay and were among the healthiest overall. The Inuit of Alaska and Canada, who consumed a very high-fat diet with negligible carbohydrate, had perfect facial bone structure and almost no dental cavities or periodontal disease. Their dental health was superior to any population he studied.

Dr. Price's findings were published in 1939 in a book titled *Nutrition and Physical Degeneration*. This book, which is still in print and currently in its eighth edition, is considered a classic in nutritional science.[4]

ARE HIGH-FAT DIETS HARMFUL?

If dietary fat was as dangerous as we have been told, then any population that eats a high-fat diet should be reeking with chronic disease and high death rates. We can easily test this hypothesis by looking at the many populations around the world that have existed for hundreds, even thousands of years on high-fat diets, and examine their health.

Most populations in the world today have adopted modern foods, sugar, refined flour, and refined vegetable oils; processed foods of all types are now available throughout the world. Even in remote villages in Bolivia, Nepal, Ethiopia, and elsewhere, modern processed foods are commonplace. But in the not-too-distant past, there were many populations around the world that thrived on traditional high-fat diets void of all modern processed foods. These people were robust and healthy, with life spans as long as ours. Let's take a look at a few of them.

British physician Dr. Hugh C. Trowell (1899-1984) worked among the primitive peoples of East Africa from 1930 to 1960. He was part of an extensive research project sponsored by the British government to study the prevalent diseases of the area. When he started his research back in 1930, the people lived as they had for thousands of years. They ate only what they foraged or killed. Except in the larger cities, Western culture had little impact on these people.

In the early years, Dr. Trowell and his coworkers noted that there was absolutely no evidence of diabetes, high blood pressure, stroke, or coronary artery disease among the people. Autopsies showed no evidence of atherosclerosis or heart disease. Over the next 30 years all that changed. Degenerative disease slowly appeared and became more prevalent over time. The natives still lived in a relative wilderness, away from industrialization, but they became increasingly dependent on white flour, sugar, and other processed foods shipped in from Western countries.

Among the natives of East Africa are a number of ethnic groups, namely, the Maasai of Tanzania and the Samburu, Rendille, and Turkana of Northern Kenya, who live a nomadic pastoral existence, tending cattle, sheep, and goats. Their diet consisted entirely of meat, milk, and on occasion, blood from their flocks. Traditionally, no vegetable products were eaten. Their diet relied heavily on raw cow's milk. Adults consumed up to 5 liters a day. This is rich, whole milk, not nonfat, so it is loaded with saturated fat and cholesterol. About 66 percent of their daily calories came from saturated fat.

Keep in mind that the American Heart Association (AHA) has counseled us that we should get no more than 30 percent of our daily calories from fat, mostly from vegetable oils, and that we should limit our intake of saturated fat to just 7 percent of total calories. Apparently, nobody bothered to inform these people about a proper diet. They were getting over 70 percent of their daily calories from fat, most of it saturated.

With this high amount of saturated fat and cholesterol, you would think these populations would all have high blood cholesterol levels and be suffering from various stages of heart disease. But they didn't, so long as they maintained their traditional high-fat diet. They did not suffer from high cholesterol, high blood pressure, atherosclerosis, or heart disease, as might be expected. In addition, diabetes, obesity, cancer, tooth decay, and other diseases of modern civilization were unknown among them.

Historically, these people depended entirely on their cattle, but in recent years maintaining a traditional pastoral lifestyle has become increasingly difficult as grazing lands have dwindled and herds have shrunk, forcing them to become more dependent on agriculture. While they still tend cattle, their diet now typically includes grains, beans, potatoes, and sugar, with far less meat and milk. Their fat intake has declined dramatically. Consequently, previously unknown diseases, such as heart disease and diabetes, are no longer strangers to them.

Coconuts, which contain a high percentage of saturated fat, are used extensively in the diet in many parts of the world. Before the introduction of Western foods, coronary heart disease was very rare among these populations.

Ian Prior, MD (1923-2009), a cardiologist and director of the epidemiology unit at the Wellington Hospital in New Zealand, led a research team during the 1960s and 1970s studying the health, diet, and lifestyle of Pacific Islanders, who traditionally consumed large quantities of coconut.

By the 1960s most Polynesian Islanders had adopted Western foods to one extent or another. Only a few populations still subsisted almost totally on their native diets. One of these populations lived on a little group of isolated islands collectively called Tokelau. This gave Prior an opportunity to study the health and diet of Polynesian Islanders with little influence from modern foods. Prior was particularly interested in how a high-fat diet, rich in coconut fat, affected the health of these people.

Tokelau consists of three small atolls in the South Pacific about 1,200 miles (2,000 km) northeast of New Zealand. In the 1960s the Tokelauans were still relatively isolated from Western influences, and the people had little interaction with non-Polynesians. Their native diet and culture remained much as it had for centuries.

Dr. Prior's studies began in the early 1960s and included the entire population of the islands. This was a long-term multidisciplinary study set up to examine the physical, social, and health consequences of migration from the atolls to New Zealand, which had jurisdiction over the islands.

Coconut palms and a few starchy tropical fruits and root vegetables supplied the vast majority of the islanders' diet, supplemented with fish, pork, and chicken. Coconuts were their major source of food. Every meal contained coconut in some form: the green nut provided the main beverage; the mature nut, grated or as coconut cream, was cooked with taro root or breadfruit; and small pieces of coconut meat made an important snack food. Plants and fish were cooked with coconut oil.

The Tokelauans were getting 57 percent of their total daily calories from fat, with 54 percent of calories as saturated fat, primarily from coconuts. They were consuming more than 1,100 calories of saturated fat each day, 17 times more than the 63-calorie limit set by the AHA.

Considering the amount of fat and saturated fat in their diet, Dr Prior and colleagues expected them to have high blood cholesterol and definite signs of heart disease. Using a formula to calculate blood cholesterol levels based on diet, Prior's team predicted they would have a total cholesterol level of nearly 300 mg/dl (7.7 mmol/l), indicating severe hypercholesterolemia (high blood cholesterol). In actuality, their cholesterol levels averaged about

210 mg/dl (5.4 mmol/l); blood cholesterol levels were about 90 mg/dl (2.3 mmol/l) lower than predicted despite the high-fat diet.

Prior reported that the islanders' overall health was excellent. There were no signs of kidney disease or hypothyroidism that might influence blood fat levels. There were no signs of hypercholesterolemia; cholesterol levels were essentially normal. All inhabitants were lean and healthy despite a very high saturated fat diet. In fact, the population as a whole had ideal weight-to-height ratios. Digestive problems were rare, and constipation uncommon. Islanders averaged two or more bowel movements a day. Atherosclerosis, heart disease, colitis, colon cancer, hemorrhoids, ulcers, diverticulosis, and appendicitis were foreign to them. "There is no evidence of the high saturated fat intake having a harmful effect in these populations," wrote Dr. Prior.

When Tokelauans migrate from their island atolls to the very different culture of New Zealand, they take on the dietary habits of their new country. Their total fat and saturated fat intake drop significantly. Processed foods take the place of much of their traditional foods. This change increases their risk of atherosclerosis and heart disease. Total cholesterol, LDL cholesterol, and triglyceride levels increase, while HDL cholesterol decreases, all unfavorable changes.

This pattern has been seen with virtually every island population as they immigrate to New Zealand, Australia, or other Western countries. "The more an Islander takes on the ways of the West, the more prone he is to succumb to our degenerative diseases," said Prior. His studies have shown that the further the Pacific natives move from the lifestyle and diet of their ancestors, "the closer they come to gout, diabetes, atherosclerosis, obesity, and hypertension."[5]

The effect of modern processed food is nowhere more dramatic than it has been on the Inuit of North America. Harvard-educated anthropologist Vilhjalmur Stefansson (1879-1962) spent much of his career studying and lecturing about the native Inuit culture of Alaska and northern Canada. Starting in 1906, he lived among the Inuit for 11 years. For most of that time he lived off the land as they did, eating caribou, fowl, musk ox, fox, fish, seal, and other wild game. He carefully recorded the types of foods the Inuit ate, noting that among the non-Westernized or primitive Inuit, their diet consisted entirely of meat and fat; they consumed no plant food whatsoever. Fat was especially relished and supplied about 80 percent of their daily calories. Special care was taken to remove all the fat from game, including the fat surrounding internal organs. None of it was wasted. All their meat was dipped in a bowl of melted seal blubber, much like a dipping sauce, before being eaten.

Did this high-fat diet harm the Inuit? Apparently not. Stefansson reported that the Inuit appeared to be immune to degenerative disease. There was

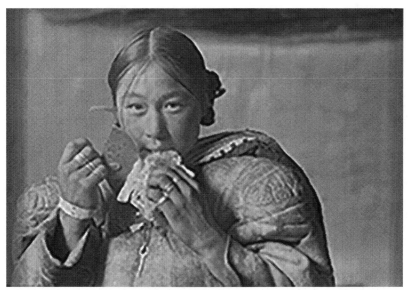
Inuit woman eating a meal of mostly fat.

no heart disease, diabetes, cancer, arthritis, or any of the diseases of modern civilization among those who lived on their ancestral, fat-based diet. The high-fat diet didn't shorten their lives either. He noted that the Inuit lived just as long as anyone in the United States or Europe at that time.

Before 1955, most Inuit lived a nomadic life, living off the land. Unless they lived in permanent settlements or near trading posts, only occasionally would they supplement their fat-based diet with store-bought foods.

Starting in the mid-1950s, the Inuit were recruited to work on military and civilian airports across the Alaskan and Canadian Arctic. By the late 1960s, almost all of the Inuit had given up their nomadic lifestyles and were living in permanent communities. They also gave up their traditional foods and began eating the same products as most North Americans—processed flour, sugar, sweets, vegetable oils, and canned goods. Before that time, the Inuit rarely ever saw sugar and never used vegetable oil. They ate caribou fat and seal blubber by the pound, but had never even tasted margarine or corn oil. These new oils took the place of the animal fats they had once eaten with relish. They started eating less meat and fat, replacing them with grains, sugar, and other processed foods.

Dr. Otto Schaefer (1919-2009), director of the Northern Medical Research Unit of the Charles Camsell Hospital in Edmonton, Canada, worked among the Inuit for more than 20 years and witnessed firsthand the transition that occurred in the 1950s and 1960s. He noted that the traditional high-fat diet was replaced with one high in sugar. In one Inuit community in the Canadian Western Arctic, he was able to get detailed records of food imports spanning eight years, from 1959 to 1967. He found that sugar consumption by the average Inuit in that area quadrupled during that time, from 26 pounds per person per year to 104.2 pounds (see table below). In 1959 sugar accounted for only 18.1 percent of the total carbohydrate they consumed. By 1967 it accounted for 44.2 percent. In 1967 each Inuit man, woman, and child, on average, consumed more than 104 pounds (47 kg) of sugar.[6] That seems like a lot, but today in the United States, we consume 130 pounds (60 kg) of sugar per person each year, in addition to the equivalent of about 20 pounds (9 kg) of sugar in the form of artificial sweeteners.

Annual Per Capita Consumption of Sugar in Pangnirtung-Cumberland Trading Area 1959-1967

Year	Per Capita (lbs/kg)	% of total Carbohydrate Consumed
1959	26/11.8	18.1
1960	37.6/17	22.4
1964	65.5/29.7	30.2
1967	104.2/47.3	44.2

Before living in permanent communities, the health of the Inuit was like most other isolated peoples. Degenerative diseases, including diabetes and heart disease, were extremely rare. Within one decade, the Inuit began experiencing degenerative disease at an alarming rate. Diabetes tripled. Dr. Schaefer noted that in this Inuit community there were more new cases of diabetes than had occurred in all of the Inuit living in all of Canada just a few years earlier.

Diabetes wasn't the only problem he saw developing among the Inuit; diseases of the arteries among men over 40 increased fivefold. Gallbladder disease skyrocketed. Cancer, which had been extremely rare among the Inuit, began to appear at an increasing rate. Even acne, which was previously unknown to the Canadian Inuit before the mid-1950s, began afflicting the youth. At one time, all of the Inuit were slim and trim even in middle age, but living in the communities, they developed bulging paunches.

With a civilized diet also came civilized disease. The Inuit had few health problems with their high-saturated fat and cholesterol diet. But as soon as they reduced their fat intake and began eating processed foods, diseases of all types, including heart disease, began to plague them. What saturated fat and cholesterol couldn't do over generations of time, sugar and white flour did in just a few years.

Other populations that thrived on high-fat diets include the Yukaghir, Chukchi, and Koryak of Siberia and the Russian Arctic, the Watusi and Bambuti of central Africa, and the San people of the Kalahari Desert. The

Somaliland camel herders subsist on nothing but camel's milk, of which they drink about a gallon each day (350 grams of animal fat). The nomadic Bedouins of the Negev desert also eat almost nothing but the fermented milk of sheep, goats, camels, and donkeys; the same is true of the Toda herders, the Dhangar caste, and the Pardhi, all pastoral tribes of India. The Ainu of northern Japan, the Finnish Lapps, the Negritos of the northern Philippine Islands, the aborigines of Australia, and the Vedda of Sri Lanka traditionally all consumed diets high in fat. Indeed, it is believed that the entire human race descended from Stone Age hunter-gatherer populations that thrived on high-fat diets. In fact, we all started life on high-fat diets as infants. Mother's milk is rich in fat and saturated fat. It is natural for us to be genetically well suited to a high-fat diet.

As you see, many populations around the world with different ethnic backgrounds not only lived but thrived on high-fat diets. The same cannot be said of sugar and refined flour. There are no traditional populations that lived primarily on sugar and white flour. These products are modern inventions that have only come into wide use over the past century. The only population that eats this way is ours, and look what is happening to us! We consume ample quantities of calories and nutrients and always have food available, but we are sicker than any generation in human history.

History has repeated itself over and over again. Whenever a people have adopted modern, processed foods, diseases of modern civilization have quickly followed. The transition from moderate- or high-fat diets to a modern low-fat, high-carb diet has always resulted in declining health. When fat is removed from the diet, it is invariably replaced with carbohydrate, so a low-fat diet is also a high-carb diet. In our modern society, these carbohydrates are primarily refined flour and sugar.

Fat is a necessary nutrient; we need it for optimal health. Sugar, and even carbohydrate in general, is not essential. Many populations thrived on diets completely devoid of all carbohydrates, yet were healthy and free from degenerative disease. Removing fat from the diet is unhealthy, as it deprives the body of essential nutrients, not just from the fat itself, but also the fat-soluble vitamins and nutrients that are only found with dietary fats.

YOU CANNOT OUTRUN A BAD DIET

When the promoters of low-fat diets are presented with the fact that many populations have thrived on high-fat diets, they claim that the reason for their good health is because these populations are also very physically active. The high level of physical activity counteracts the negative effects of the high-fat diet. If a high-fat diet with as much as 80 percent of calories from fat is not harmful when combined with daily physical activity, then this would mean that diet has a rather minor effect on health in comparison to exercise. This is to say that physical activity is vastly more important to our overall health than diet. Is that true? We know that exercise is important for good health and well-being, but can it actually prevent or reverse heart disease, diabetes, cancer, and other degenerative diseases regardless of diet?

While many people are woefully sedentary, a large portion of the population is exercising more now than ever before. Fitness clubs and gym memberships are at all-time highs. Exercise equipment and workout videos are among the hottest-selling products. Endurance sports, such as marathon running, cycling, and triathlons, are much more common now than in years past. Yet the fitness trend has not stopped the rising rates of diabetes and obesity. If exercise were the key ingredient to good health, then athletes, particularly marathon runners and other endurance athletes would be totally immune to heart disease and other chronic illnesses. But they aren't. Athletes suffer from heart attacks, strokes, diabetes, and other chronic illnesses just like everybody else.

A prime example of this is fitness expert James Fixx, the author of the 1977 best-selling book *The Complete Book of Running*. Fixx was an outspoken advocate of the health benefits of exercise, claiming that active people live longer, and was one of the primary forces behind the popularization of jogging. He ran several miles daily and was a lean, muscular 159 pounds. He competed in numerous Boston Marathons and won the Connecticut 10,000-meter championship in his age category. He was declared medically fitter than most college athletes. Yet, he died of a massive heart attack while jogging at the relatively youthful age of 52. An autopsy revealed that he had extensive atherosclerosis, with coronary arteries that were as much as 95 percent blocked. His arteries looked more like those of an 85-year-old.

Fixx is not a rare case of a physically fit person succumbing to degenerative disease. Many relatively young athletes die each year from heart attacks, strokes, cancer, and other diseases. Although more physically fit than the average person, they are not immune to degenerative disease. There have been numerous cases of highly trained marathon runners dying from heart disease. In one study, 36 cases were analyzed. The mean age of the athletes was 43.8 years; the youngest was only 18 when he died. The mean number of years they had been training and competing in marathons was 6.8.[7] Getting regular exercise and being physically fit did not protect them from heart disease. The claim that physical activity is what protects primitive cultures from heart disease and other chronic health problems regardless of their diet, doesn't hold up.

Of the 36 athletes in the study who died from heart disease, not one of them ate a high-fat diet. They ate a low-fat, high-carb diet with lean protein—the diet that has been generally recommended for optimal health and good physical performance. Carbohydrate is our bodies' primary source of fuel to produce energy, and protein is needed to build strong muscles. Fat is considered a more or less useless nutrient that just crowds out the more desired carbohydrate and protein, so the less fat eaten, the better. Most top-notch endurance athletes practice carbohydrate loading, which is to load up on high-carb foods such as bread, pasta, cake, cookies, and pancakes for several days before competition or a heavy workout. This is done to store up as much glucose as the body can hold to provide the energy needed for maximum endurance. Despite eating a low-fat diet and being in excellent physical shape, these athletes still died from degenerative heart disease. It was likely the low-fat, high-carb diet that killed them.

Peter Attia, MD, a physician who specializes in preventative medicine, knows personally that exercise alone will not prevent or reverse chronic disease. Peter is a dedicated endurance athlete working out 3 to 4 hours daily. He is one of only a dozen people to swim the Catalina Channel off the coast of Southern California in both directions (on separate occasions), a distance of 21 miles (34 km) each way—the same distance as swimming the English Channel. He has also crossed the Maui channel, swimming from Maui to Lanai and back—a distance of 20 miles (32 km).

Despite his hours of daily exercise and highly fit physical condition, he found his health gradually declining. He was getting chubby. In high school he weighed 160 pounds (72.5 kg). At age 35 and at peak physical condition, he weighed a pudgy 195 pounds and carried about 40 pounds of body fat. He was fit but fat. He was also developing insulin resistance, the hallmark feature of type 2 diabetes. He had three of the five markers for metabolic syndrome—a group of symptoms that indicate an increased risk of heart disease, diabetes, and other chronic conditions. He ate what he believed at the time was a healthy high-carb, low-fat diet, never ate at fast-food restaurants, and avoided junk foods. However, his intense exercise could not overcome the negative effects of his supposedly healthy low-fat diet.

Peter is very conscious about his health and carefully monitors what he eats. In 2009 he was consuming a total of 3,170 calories per day, consisting of 600 grams of carbohydrate, 200 grams of protein, and 50 grams of fat. A mere 14 percent of his daily calories came from fat, while 64 percent came from carbohydrate. In most people's view this would be considered an ideal diet for a physically active person.

Yet despite this "healthy" low-fat diet, he was on the path toward chronic disease. Exercise wasn't solving the problem. He decided to focus more on his diet. He started by cutting out most sources of sugar and replacing refined grains and flours with whole grains. These changes brought a noticeable improvement, which encouraged him to further refine his diet by eliminating all sugar and reducing total carbohydrate intake to fewer than 50 grams per day. Protein was also reduced to about 120 grams per day, and fat consumption increased to 425 grams daily.

Over a two-year period Peter gradually adopted a very low-carb, high-fat diet—a ketogenic diet. He was consuming 1,200 calories more each day than he had before, with 88 percent of those calories coming from fat, mostly saturated fat. Even though he was consuming more total calories and an enormous amount of fat, he lost weight and dropped from 20 percent body fat to 7.5 percent, his waist circumference shrank from 38 to 32 inches (96 to 81 cm), his LDL cholesterol fell from 113 to 59 mg/dl, triglycerides dropped from 154 to 81 mg/dl, and HDL cholesterol (the so-called good cholesterol that protects against heart disease) increased from 31 to 85 mg/dl. The amount of time he spent exercising decreased by about an hour each day, but his exercise performance significantly improved. All aspects of his health improved dramatically on this new low-carb, high-fat diet.

Dr. Attia has maintained a low-carb, high-fat diet since 2011. He is no longer overweight or insulin resistant and enjoys exceptional health. He now lectures throughout the world about the health benefits of the ketogenic diet. You can visit his website at www.eatingacademy.com.

Low-fat, high-carb diets are generally overloaded with refined flour and sugar and are not healthy. Getting plenty of exercise does not prevent heart disease, diabetes, overweight, or other chronic health problems if the diet is poor. No amount of running or exercise will protect you from a bad diet. Likewise, regular physical activity is not the magic bullet that protects primitive societies from degenerative disease. It is the sugar-free diet that does that.

3

The War On Fat

THE HEART DISEASE EPIDEMIC

Our ancient hunter-gatherer ancestors were largely carnivorous, with a hunger for fat. They would eat every morsel of fat on their prey, including the fat surrounding the internal organs, and even crack open the bones to get at the fatty marrow inside. In cooler climates hunter-gatherer societies subsisted almost entirely on meat and fat. In warmer regions primitive peoples had greater access to plant foods and consequently ate less meat and fat. In both cases, however, the most common source of fat was of animal origin. Throughout history the human body was well adapted to eating and thriving on diets rich in saturated fat and cholesterol. It is unlikely that humans could have existed all this time if we had been eating a diet that caused heart disease, diabetes, and other conditions that led to ill health and premature death.

Saturated fat and cholesterol have been a part of the human diet for as long as we have been around. The idea that they are harmful doesn't make any sense historically. So, how did saturated fat become the evil villain it is known as today?

Heart disease is an affliction of modern society. In primitive cultures, both ancient and modern, it is extremely rare. There were no recorded cases of this illness in the medical literature until the latter half of the 19th century. The first documented case of a person suffering a heart attack was published in Britain in 1878. Dr. Adam Hammer reported the unusual case of a patient who experienced crushing chest pain, then collapsed and died. An autopsy found that muscle tissue in the patient's heart had died, resulting in heart failure and death. Nowadays, the signs of heart attack are well-known and common. Thousands of people die every day. But a century ago it was almost unheard-of.

31

The advancement of medicine took a giant leap forward during the 19th century. From 1830 to 1880 most of the diseases that plagued mankind at the time were identified and named. In Europe autopsies became routine. Tens of thousands of autopsies were performed during this time to accelerate the advance of the science of medicine. Much of our current knowledge of anatomy, physiology, and pathology developed at this time. During this period, not a single heart attack was recorded until 1878. Nowadays, heart attack is the most common cause of death.

Some people might claim that heart disease wasn't recorded before that time because the doctors of that period didn't know what the disease looked like. In other words, they were too ignorant to know what they were looking at. This argument isn't valid because these "old-time" doctors were the ones who identified the signs of the disease that are used today. Also, there were many doctors who lived during the era of transition into modern medicine who saw firsthand the changes that occurred in the human body over time.

Dr. Paul Dudley White is known as the founder of American cardiology—the study of the heart and its diseases. He graduated from medical school in 1910 and served as President Dwight D. Eisenhower's personal physician during his terms in office. As a young man, White wrote that he had an interest in a rare new disease that he had read about in the European medical literature. It was 1921, 11 years after he began his practice, when he saw his first heart attack patient. At that time, heart attacks were extremely rare.[1]

From 1910 to 1920 heart disease deaths in the United States were very low, affecting only about 10 out of every 100,000 people per year. By 1930 the death rate jumped to 46 per 100,000, and by 1970 the rate reached 331 per 100,000.

In the early 1950s heart disease became the number one killer in the United States, Canada, Australia, and much of Europe. Medical researchers frantically sought for the elusive cause of this new epidemic.

One of the biggest changes that occurred from 1910 to 1950 was the dramatic changes in the diet. Apparently, the diet might have something to do with this new epidemic. Researchers wondered, what was it in the Western diet that could cause such a rapid degeneration of health?

The disease seemed to be connected to affluence. The questions researchers asked were, "What are the characteristic features of the diets of wealthy populations? Are there some dietary features that have changed which parallel the great increase in wealth in the countries of Western Europe and North America?" And, "How do the diets of poor populations differ from those of wealthy populations?"

To answer these questions, researchers analyzed the diets of the affluent and the poor and compared them with coronary heart disease statistics.

When the foods eaten by people in the poorest countries were compared with those in the wealthiest, researchers found that the latter ate 50 percent more calories, which were derived from 70 percent more protein and four or five times more fat. The amount of total carbohydrate consumed was not much different. Micronutrients, such as the types of fat or carbohydrate consumed, were not analyzed.

From this data the most dramatic change was in the increased consumption of protein and particularly fat. Consequently, in the 1950s researchers began focusing their attention on dietary fat as the possible cause of coronary heart disease.

THE CHOLESTEROL HYPOTHESIS

In 1953, Ancel Keys, PhD, then director of the Laboratory of Physiological Hygiene at the University of Minnesota, wrote a paper that appeared to give credence to the idea that fat was the primary culprit behind the heart disease epidemic.[2] His proof was based on a graph that showed a close correction between total fat intake and death rates from coronary heart disease in six seemingly random countries (Japan, Italy, England/Wales, Australia, Canada, and the United States). The points on the graph form an almost perfect parabolic curve, something that is more like what you would get with a physics experiment rather than in biology. If the curve were to extend farther to the right, it would shoot almost straight upward, indicating that a diet of 50 percent or more of calories from fat was a certain death sentence from heart disease. Extending the curve to the left indicated that a diet devoid of all fat would impart total immunity from ever experiencing a heart attack. The data looked convincing, to say the least.

Keys later refined his idea, stating that saturated fats rather than all fats are the real culprit, and he proposed what is now known as the *diet-heart hypothesis*, also known as the lipid or cholesterol hypothesis. According to Keys, the consumption of saturated fat and cholesterol raises blood cholesterol levels. The higher the blood cholesterol, the more likely some of it will adhere to the artery walls in the form of arterial plaque, causing atherosclerosis. As plaque builds up, it could block the flow of blood and oxygen in a coronary artery feeding the heart, causing a heart attack, or in a carotid artery feeding the brain, causing a stroke.

Keys based his new theory in part on a study published 40 years earlier by Russian scientist Nikolai Anichkov. Anichkov fed cholesterol to rabbits and found that they developed atherosclerotic plaques similar, but not identical, to those found in humans.

Since cholesterol was the primary fat identified in human arterial plaque, it was assumed that cholesterol was the villain. Scientists, although they did

33

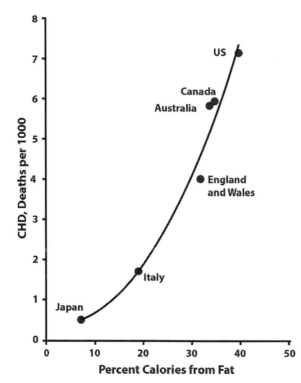

Ancel Keys's Six Countries study plotted heart disease deaths for men aged 55-59 years of age from data supplied by the Food and Agriculture Organization of the United Nations (FAO) for the years 1948-1949.

not understand how, theorized that cholesterol accumulated in the arterial walls gives rise to the plaque deposits characteristic of atherosclerosis and, consequently, leads to heart disease. It was reasoned that the more cholesterol that is in the blood, the more likely some of it will be deposited in the arteries. This led to the assumption that a diet high in cholesterol and saturated fat (which the body can convert to cholesterol) caused heart attacks and strokes. This theory provided a simple answer to a perplexing problem.

The cholesterol hypothesis was immediately hailed as the long-sought-for cause of heart disease. Many doctors were quick to accept the new hypothesis, as it provided a seemingly logical and convenient answer to the heart disease mystery. Representatives from the American Heart Association appeared on television to warn people about the dangers of eating too much butter, lard, eggs, and red meats. Keys wrote a book titled *Eat Well and Stay Well* in 1959 to further convince the medical community and the general public of his diet-heart hypothesis. Keys received wide acclaim and was honored by *Time* magazine on January 13, 1961, which featured an article about his "discovery" and pictured him on the front cover.

FLAWS IN KEYS'S HYPOTHESIS

Despite the rapid acceptance of Keys's hypothesis, not all scientists were convinced. Paul Dudley White, MD, the foremost authority in the United States on cardiology and, consequently, heart disease, at the time stated that he couldn't support the diet-heart hypothesis because he knew it didn't fit the history of the disease. People had been eating saturated fat for generations without it causing any harm; why suddenly would it cause harm now? Also, saturated fat consumption had been declining over the previous 30 years, at the very same time heart disease was increasing. It just didn't make any sense. If heart disease was caused by something in the diet, it had to be something that wasn't eaten, or eaten as often in previous generations as it was then.

Researchers Jacob Yerushalmy and Herman Hilleboe took another look at Keys's data and discovered something amiss. Keys had diet and heart disease death data available to him for 22 countries, but he only plotted six. Why would he ignore the vast majority of his data to prove his theory? You would think that if his hypothesis were correct, the complete data would provide a far more accurate and convincing argument. When Yerushalmy and Hilleboe used the data from all 22 countries and replotted Keys's graph, a curious thing happened: the perfect correlation between fat and heart disease was no longer so perfect. In fact, the correlation almost completely disappeared. Some countries with high fat consumption had much lower heart disease rates than those with low fat intakes. For example, fat consumption in Finland was seven times that of Mexico, but the two countries had similar heart disease death rates.[3]

The apparent correlation between fat intake and heart disease didn't completely disappear with the addition of the missing data, but it was significantly reduced, making Keys's argument less convincing. It must be pointed out that correlation does not equate to causation, meaning that simply because there is a correlation between two variables, it does not mean that one causes the other. If correlations did prove causation, you could make some ridiculous conclusions. For example, since the 1950s both atmospheric CO_2 levels and obesity levels have increased sharply. Therefore, you might conclude that atmospheric CO_2 causes obesity. However, further research needs to be conducted to positively link the two variables. In this case, the real reason for the correlation is that richer populations tend to eat more food and produce more CO_2. There was no direct cause-and-effect relationship between the two, but both were affected by a third variable—prosperity. You always have to be careful with correlations.

While Keys focused his attention on the correlation between heart disease deaths and fats, his data also contained information on other fac-

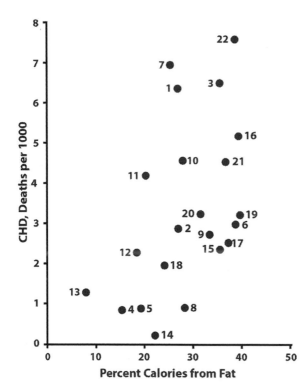

Using the data from all 22 countries for men 55-59 years of age from the FAO for the years 1951-1953. 1. Australia, 2. Italy, 3. Canada, 4. Ceylon, 5. Chile, 6. Denmark, 7 Finland, 8. France, 9 West Germany, 10. Ireland, 11. Israel, 12. Italy, 13, Japan, 14. Mexico, 15. Holland, 16. New Zealand, 17. Norway, 18. Portugal, 19. Sweden, 20. Switzerland, 21. Great Britain, 22. USA. Data from Yerushalmy and Hilleboe

tors, such as smoking and protein and sugar consumption. Yerushalmy and Hilleboe calculated the correlation coefficients of each. The correlation coefficient tells how well two variables are related to each other. A coefficient of 1 indicates the strongest possible correlation. A coefficient of 0 indicates the weakest or no correlation. Using data from all 22 countries, the correlation coefficient of heart disease deaths and fat consumption turned out to be 0.56, indicating only a slight relationship. However, the correlation coefficient with sugar was 0.68, indicating a much stronger relationship. Cigarette smoking, which is now regarded as a major risk factor for heart disease, had a coefficient of 0.64, indicating a closer relationship to heart disease than fat but not as close as sugar. Why did Keys ignore this stronger relationship with sugar in preference to fat?

Keys, it turned out, carefully selected the data that he used to purposely design a graph that would give the impression that dietary fat was closely related to heart disease deaths. The study was seriously flawed, yet it was one of the most crucial studies in convincing the majority of the scientific community that fat was the primary cause of heart disease.

THE FAT VERSUS SUGAR DEBATE
The Case Against Sugar

A number of researchers suspected sugar to be a more likely culprit behind the heart disease epidemic. The most prominent among them was John Yudkin, MD, PhD, a physician and biochemist and a distinguished professor of nutrition at Queen Elizabeth College of the University of London.

The rise in sugar consumption in affluent countries during the early 20th century closely mirrored the rise in heart disease. Although this was only a correlation and didn't prove sugar was the cause, it led Yudkin and others to investigate the relationship in more detail.

Dietary fat was first scrutinized as a possible contributing factor in the growing rate of heart disease because fat consumption was much higher in affluent countries, while total carbohydrate consumption was about the same. The effects of the different types of carbohydrate weren't generally recognized at the time, so sugar wasn't seriously considered. However, there was a dramatic change in the type of carbohydrate consumed in affluent countries. Complex carbohydrates from whole grains and vegetables were replaced by refined flour and sugar. While the vast majority of total calories in people's diets continued to come from carbohydrate, the type of carbohydrate changed from the traditional to the highly processed. Carbohydrate today typically accounts for 50 to 60 percent of a person's total calorie intake. If only half of that is changed from complex carbohydrates to sugar and refined flour, that is a huge amount of nutritionally empty calories added to the diet and a loss of a significant amount of nutrition. In the United States, for example, sugar consumption nearly doubled from 1909 to 1999, yet during the same period total fat intake increased by a mere one-eighth. The type of fat changed too: vegetable oil intake *increased* while animal fat consumption *decreased*, which was assumed to be a healthy transition even though heart disease rates continued to rise as animal fat consumption declined.

The history of heart disease suggests a stronger link with sugar consumption than with saturated fat. Yudkin pointed out that there were several groups, such as the Samburu and Maasai peoples of East Africa and the tribesmen of Mongolia, who ate a tremendous amount of animal fat, but no sugar, and they were completely immune to heart disease. When they added processed flour and sugar into their diets and even reduced the amount of fat, they become susceptible to heart disease. In similar fashion, the increased use of sugar in the UK and other affluent countries paralleled the rise in heart disease. In the United Kingdom toward the latter end of the 19th century, Britons consumed an average of 25 pounds (11 kg) of sugar each per year, heart disease was almost unheard of. By the 1970s the amount of sugar had increased to 120 pounds (54 kg), and heart disease had grown to be the number one killer. Yet total carbohydrate consumption remained about the same. In every instance throughout the world, as sugar consumption increased, so did heart disease and other diseases of modern civilization. This pattern had been seen over and over again without a single exception.

Yudkin found the association with sugar was stronger than between cholesterol or saturated fat.[4] For example, in one study, Yudkin and his team used subjects who had suffered a nonfatal heart attack but had never had any heart problems before their initial incident. The investigators collected food consumption data on each of them before the attack. They found that compared to men with no history of heart disease, those who suffered heart attacks had been consuming substantially more sugar.[5]

By the late 1960s several studies had been done in an attempt to verify the cholesterol hypothesis. Subjects were asked to change their diet with the goal of reducing their chances of experiencing a heart attack. This was done in two ways; with a group of apparently healthy people, to see if they could prevent heart attack, and with a group of people who had had one or more attacks, to see if they could prevent having another attack. The results were mixed. In those studies that reported the highest correlation with saturated fat reduction, Yudkin pointed out that they also simultaneously reduced sugar consumption, so the results could have just as well have been from the lower sugar intake.

Many studies that appeared to point a critical finger at fat could have equally implicated sugar. For example, a study reported from Oslo, Norway in 1967 used subjects who had already had one or more heart attacks. In this study, the dietary instructions were not simply to limit saturated fat, but also sugary foods, such as candy, cakes, cookies, and ice cream. As a result, the intake of sugar, as well as saturated fat, was considerably reduced.[6] However, the reduction in fat was spotlighted as the primary concern.

Another incidence reported in 1958 involved patients from two mental hospitals in Finland. One hospital replaced the butter and the butterfat in milk they ordinarily used with highly unsaturated vegetable fats. The other hospital, which served as the control, maintained their normal servings of butter and whole-fat milk. It turned out, however, that throughout the trial, the diet in the experimental hospital contained only about half the amount of sugar as was used in the diet of the control hospital. Of course, the lower cardiac events were attributed to the reduced fat content, and not the reduced sugar. Were these omissions about the contribution of sugar to the study's results done on purpose or just sloppy research?

Unfortunately, not all studies report sugar consumption, perhaps because the investigators at the time did not bother to distinguish between the types of carbohydrate subjects consumed. Overlooking the sugar content of the experimental diets could render these studies worthless, making the results of some of the older studies that helped fuel the cholesterol hypothesis questionable.

In the 1950s most medical researchers held to the belief that the body handles all dietary carbohydrate in the same way. Since the total intake of carbohydrate was no higher in countries where heart disease was prevalent than it was in those where it was less prevalent, it was not deemed worthwhile to consider dietary carbohydrate or its constituent parts as possible causes of coronary heart disease.

Epidemiologic studies by Yudkin and others in the 1950s and 1960s showed that sugar has the highest correlation of any component of the diet, including saturated fat and cholesterol, with the incidence of coronary artery disease.[7-9]

B. K. Armstrong and colleagues looked at the correlation between ischemic heart disease mortality and commodity consumption in 30 countries in the years 1963-1965. They found sugar to have the strongest correlation, even stronger than saturated fat, total fat, or cigarettes.[10] The scientific community seemed to ignore these studies.

Much of Yudkin's research in the 1960s was devoted to learning what happens when we replace the complex carbohydrates in our diet with sugar. He found that the replacement of complex carbohydrates with sucrose, in proportions no greater than what is typically consumed, produces a large number of very profound metabolic changes.

Saturated fat was condemned because it had a tendency to raise blood cholesterol levels. Yudkin found that dietary sugar could have an equal effect on raising blood cholesterol and a greater effect on triglyceride levels than saturated fat. Some saturated fats, it was later discovered, such as stearic acid found in beef, and capric and caprylic acids found in tropical oils, had little or no effect on blood cholesterol.

In several animal species sugar stunted their growth. According to Yudkin, this was not due primarily to the decrease in nutrition, but to less efficient utilization of the nutrients in the animals' diet. The activities of many enzymes are also changed, which could result in fatty liver disease and kidney damage. Sugar is readily fermentable by oral bacteria that live in dental plaque and contribute to tooth decay. The ingestion of sugar causes rapid changes in blood glucose levels, with nefarious metabolic effects, including damage to artery walls, which promotes the development of atherosclerosis. It didn't take huge amounts of sugar to cause these changes. Many of them were demonstrated with diets containing proportions of sugar that were no higher than those found in the diet at the time and were accepted as normal.

One of Yudkin's greatest concerns was sugar's effect on insulin levels. By the 1960s, there was considerable evidence linking type 2 diabetes and coronary heart disease. Diabetics are prone to develop heart disease, and people with heart disease are generally found to be overt or latent diabetics, or at least to have impaired glucose tolerance (insulin resistance).

A number of other observations link diabetes and heart disease to high insulin levels. First, hyperinsulinism (high insulin levels) is found in both diseases, even if there is no evidence of the other disease.

Second, hyperinsulinism is also found in peripheral vascular disease, in hypertension, and in obesity, conditions that are known to be associated with coronary heart disease. Smoking is also known to cause hyperinsulinism, while physical exercise, which is protective against coronary disease, reduces the level of blood insulin.

Third, injection of insulin in rats was shown to increase the deposition of plaque in the arteries of the aorta. In young roosters, carbutamide (which stimulates insulin) increased spontaneous atherosclerosis.

In a clinical study, Yudkin found that six out of nineteen apparently healthy men developed hyperinsulinism after 14 days on a sucrose-rich diet. Sucrose ingestion thus fell into line with diabetes, peripheral vascular disease, smoking, hypertension, and physical activity. These conditions are generally recognized as affecting an individual's proneness to atherosclerotic disease; all are known to affect insulin levels.

Yudkin claimed, "If only a small fraction of what we know about the effects of sugar were to be revealed in relation to any other material used as a food additive, that material would promptly be banned." Yet, the harshest warning the public received about sugar was "don't eat too much,' primarily because it may promote cavities.

The War On Fat Heats Up

Ancel Keys and John Yudkin clashed with their competing theories. The only thing that prevented the fat hypothesis from universal acceptance was Yudkin's determined insistence that sugar was the culprit and not fat. Keys was charismatic, combative, and critical to the point of skewering his opponents. He was intensely critical of Yudkin and the sugar hypothesis. When Yudkin published a paper, Keys would berate it and would attack him personally as an inept dupe, saying that the "evidence" Yudkin had presented would "not bear up under the most elementary critical examination." He called Yudkin's theory "a mountain of nonsense." And he accused Yudkin of issuing "propaganda" for the meat and dairy industries. "Yudkin and his commercial backers are not deterred by the facts," he said. "They continue to sing the same discredited tune." Keys tried to discredit Yudkin by depicting him as a patsy for the meat and dairy industries, which was ironic since Keys's primary financial backer was the sugar industry.

Yudkin, on the other hand, never responded in like manner. He was a mild-mannered academic and preferred to avoid conflict, choosing to combat Keys with science rather than rhetoric and innuendos. Unfortunately, that made him vulnerable to Keys's attacks as well as attacks from other nutritionists in Keys's camp, and from the sugar industry, which referred to Yudkin's work as "science fiction."

Keys was determined to destroy Yudkin's reputation in an all-out effort to promote his own theory. As a result, Yudkin's career never recovered. Yudkin became frustrated in his attempts to inform colleagues and the public of his findings. Few in the medical community would listen to him even though he had hard scientific evidence to back him up. Research journals stopped accepting his papers for publication. He was unwelcome at nutrition conferences. It became common to have entire conferences canceled if his name was listed as a speaker.

In 1971, at age 61, Yudkin relinquished his position at the University of London to devote full time to writing a book for the lay readership detailing his case against sugar. In 1972, *Pure, White and Deadly* was published. The book summarized the evidence that the overconsumption of sugar greatly increased the incidence of coronary heart disease, and that it was involved in dental caries, obesity, diabetes, and liver disease, and possibly gout, dyspepsia, and some cancers. By the time he wrote his book, however, public opinion had swung completely in Keys's favor and the cholesterol hypothesis was enshrined in the dietary recommendations of professional health and medical associations. Yudkin's book got little notice.

In the mid-1950s Keys began recruiting collaborating researchers outside the United States to gather data on middle-aged men to examine the relationships between lifestyle, diet, coronary heart disease, and stroke in different populations and regions of the world. This was the world's first multinational, multiyear epidemiological study. Known as the Seven Countries Study, it included 16 cohort populations comprising more than 12,000 healthy men ages 40 to 59 in seven countries, who were followed for more than 15 years. It was first published in 1978, with follow-up studies appearing periodically in later years. Not surprisingly, the study showed a correlation between the intake of saturated fats and deaths from heart disease, just as Keys predicted. This study sealed the coffin on Yudkin's career and put to rest any lingering doubts about saturated fats being involved in heart disease. It also removed sugar from the suspect list. The cholesterol hypothesis was now firmly established in the scientific community. The debate was over.

The Seven Countries Study included data from carefully chosen populations living in the United States, Netherlands, Finland, Italy, Yugoslavia, Greece, and Japan. A question one might ask is why did Keys choose these particular populations in these particular countries? Conspicuously missing were data from countries such as France and Germany, which had high animal fat consumption but low rates of heart disease. It looks like Keys was up to his old tricks again, carefully selecting data from populations that would give the outcome he wanted.

Other influential researchers joined Keys in the battle against saturated fat; most notably Fredrick Stare and Mark Hegsted. Stare founded the Department of Nutrition at the Harvard School of Public Health in 1942 and served as its chairman for 34 years before retiring in 1976. He was the founding editor of *Nutrition Reviews*, wrote a nationally syndicated column for many years entitled "Food and Your Health," and published several popular books on nutrition. Stare was a member of the scientific advisory committee of the Sugar Research Foundation—the research arm of the sugar industry. Stare coauthored a report with Keys, which recommended replacing saturated fats with polyunsaturated fats as a means of lowering cholesterol to reduce the risk of heart attacks and strokes.[11] This advice eventually led to the disproportionate consumption of polyunsaturated oils (rich in omega-6 fats) in relation to omega-3 fats and to a general universal imbalance in the omega-6/omega-3 ratio (see Chapter 7).

Mark Hegsted, another faculty member at the Harvard School of Public Health, served on the editorial board of the most influential nutrition journals: *Journal of Lipid Research*, *Nutrition Reviews*, *American Journal of Clinical Nutrition*, and *Journal of Nutrition* and helped draft the first edition of *Dietary Guidelines for Americans*. A significant part of American nutrition policy was shaped by Stare and Hegsted.

In the aftermath, Yudkin's scientific reputation was ruined. Yudkin had become an embarrassment to the University of London, an eccentric who could not accept the path that modern nutritional science was headed. After retirement, the university reneged on a promise to allow him to continue to use its research facilities. A new researcher, who fully supported the fat hypothesis, was hired to replace him. The university was eager to shed itself of Yudkin and all ties to his foolish theory. The man who had founded and built the nutrition department for the university found himself unwelcome. He was forced to get aid from a solicitor to settle the disagreement. Eventually, the university allowed him to use a small room in a building separated from the nutrition department. Yudkin died in 1995, his legacy tarnished and his work on sugar largely forgotten.

John Yudkin had distinguished himself as one of the world's leading nutritionists. Yet, his clash with Keys and the sugar industry destroyed his career and reputation. Other researchers at the time who witnessed what happened to Yudkin, didn't want the same thing to happen to them, so they avoided doing research on sugar and focused their efforts on the politically acceptable diet-heart hypothesis.

Ancel Keys coauthored with his wife three books, two of which became bestsellers: *Eat Well and Stay Well* (1959), *The Benevolent Bean* (1967), and *How to Eat Well and Stay Well the Mediterranean Way* (1975).

Payouts from the sugar industry and royalties from his books provided him enough wealth to build an extravagant villa on the Mediterranean coast of southern Italy, known as Minnelea, where he retired in peaceful luxury. He lived there for most of the remainder of his life.

Unfavorable Results Ignored

Keys's cholesterol hypothesis was based on the concept that high blood cholesterol was the underlying cause of atherosclerosis and heart disease. Ironically, his own studies disproved this hypothesis.

Before proposing the cholesterol hypothesis, in a 1952 study Keys showed that serum cholesterol is not a valid indicator of heart disease risk. In this paper he demonstrated that there was a natural tendency in healthy men for cholesterol levels to increase with age. His data showed that at age 20, healthy males have a serum cholesterol level of around 190 mg/dl (4.9 mmol/l), which increases to more than 260 mg/dl (6.7 mmol/l) by age 70.[12] His own studies showed that cholesterol levels were affected more by age than by diet. After he proposed the cholesterol hypothesis, he never mentioned this study, completely ignoring it as if it never existed.

Keys was aware that his Seven Countries Study was only an observational study and that proof of his hypothesis required evidence of causality. For this reason, he set out to publish what was to be a major landmark study where the diet of the test subjects could be carefully controlled and provide the solid proof he was seeking. The study known as the Minnesota Coronary Experiment was conducted from 1968 to 1973. This was a tightly controlled, double-blind, randomized controlled clinical trial that analyzed the diets and health outcomes of more than 9,400 people at six state mental hospitals and a nursing home. The study was paid for by the National Heart, Lung and Blood Institute and led by Dr. Ivan Frantz, a close colleague of Keys at the University of Minnesota.

Many diet studies have relied on the participants' recalling what they ate over previous days or weeks. Such studies are limited by the accuracy of the subjects' memories, and therefore, are not totally reliable. This study was significant because the researchers knew precisely what the participants ate because the meals were prepared in the institutions' kitchens and carefully controlled. Half of the subjects were fed meals rich in saturated fats from milk, cheese, and beef. The remaining group ate a diet in which most of the saturated fat was removed and replaced with corn oil—a polyunsaturated fat. The study also had the benefit of detailed autopsies on 149 patients who had

43

died during the study. The investigation was intended to show that removing saturated fat from people's diets and replacing it with polyunsaturated vegetable oil would lower blood cholesterol and thus protect them against heart disease and lower their risk of mortality.

The saturated fats-heart disease connection had never been demonstrated in a randomized controlled trial, and this study was meant to prove Keys's hypothesis. This study was conducted at the same time that Keys was coordinating the Seven Countries Study and would have provided powerful validation of the cholesterol hypothesis and the dangers of saturated fat.

Unfortunately, after spending hundreds of thousands of dollars and several years conducting the research, Keys never published the full results of this study. In 1989, more than a decade and a half after the conclusion of the study, Keys's colleague, Ivan Frantz, published a partial analysis of the data. This paper concluded with a statement suggesting the results were essentially inconclusive: "For the entire study population, no differences between the treatment (high linoleic acid group) and control (high saturated fat group) were observed for cardiovascular events, cardiovascular deaths, or total mortality."[13] The study made no noticeable impact and was soon forgotten. Interestingly, there was no mention of Keys's involvement in the study. He had completely distanced himself from the work that was meant to prove his hypothesis. Despite being one of the largest tightly controlled clinical dietary trials of its kind ever conducted, the complete data were never fully analyzed, and consequently never published. Why put so much effort and expense into a study and not publish it?

Christopher E. Ramsden, a medical investigator at the National Institutes of Health, learned about the long-overlooked study. Intrigued, he contacted the University of Minnesota in hopes of reviewing the unpublished data. Dr. Ivan Frantz had died in 2009, but Ramsden was able to contact his son, who found the data among his father's papers hidden away in his basement, and turned it over to Ramsden for analysis.

The results were a surprise. Participants who ate a diet low in saturated fat and enriched with corn oil reduced their cholesterol by an average of 14 percent. But the low-saturated fat diet did not reduce mortality. In fact, the study found that the greater the drop in cholesterol, the higher the risk of death during the trial.

The fact that blood cholesterol levels decreased when corn oil replaced the saturated fat was expected, as this had been observed before. What wasn't expected was that the drop in cholesterol was correlated with an increase in the number of deaths. The findings ran counter to Keys's hypothesis. This study revealed just the opposite and provided strong evidenced discrediting Keys's cholesterol hypothesis. In was no wonder that Keys disavowed any involvement with the study and that the complete analysis was never published.

The new analysis of the Minnesota Coronary data was eventually published in the April 2016 edition of the *British Medical Journal,* some 40 years after the study was completed.[14] Based on the analysis, the authors concluded that although the replacement of polyunsaturated vegetable oils for saturated fat in the diet can lower total blood cholesterol, it does not lower the risk of death from coronary heart disease or any other cause. Cholesterol levels do not accurately predict coronary heart disease risk. Keys's ignored 1952 study was correct, total cholesterol is affected more by age than by diet.

The Sugar Conspiracy

The attack on Yudkin spearheaded by Keys was not simply an act of professional rivalry, but a carefully orchestrated scheme to discredit Yudkin and his theory. The sugar industry had been funding Keys's work since the early 1940s. Keys was a respected researcher whom they knew well and trusted to promote their agenda. Through Keys, the sugar industry succeeded in diverting suspicion away from sugar as a possible cause of heart disease and placing the blame squarely on saturated fat.

Buying the loyalty of respected researchers and producing studies favorable to the sugar industry were only part of the sugar industry's multipronged marketing campaign to win over the medical community and the general public.

In the 1940s the sugar industry became concerned about the general belief that sugar could possibly be contributing to a number of health problems, such as tooth decay and diabetes. In 1943 the Sugar Research Foundation (later renamed the Sugar Association) was founded to build a coalition of all of the major sugar companies and growers throughout the United States. A subsidiary was formed called Sugar Information Inc., to spearhead their public relations campaign.

In 1968 the Sugar Association, in an effort to enlist foreign sugar companies and strengthen their financial position and influence, created a research division called the International Sugar Research Foundation (ISRF). The ISRF was created to fund research to counter, as they put it, "misconceptions concerning the causes of tooth decay, diabetes, and heart problems." In time, the Sugar Association opened its doors of membership to snack and beverage companies such as Coca-Cola, Hershey's, General Mills, and Nabisco, to help bankroll their marketing campaign.

If it wasn't for the unrelenting efforts of Cristin Kearns, DDS, much of the information about the sugar industry's clandestine involvement in the saturated fat debate may have never come to light. Kearns worked as a dental health administrator for Kaiser Permanente's Dental Care Program. As part of her job, she attended the 2007 annual conference of the Institute for Oral Health. The focus of that year's conference was on the links between diabetes and gum disease.

Conference speakers instructed attendees about healthy food choices for their diabetic patients. The recommendations, however, didn't seem right. As the dental director for low-income clinics in Denver, Kearns had seen firsthand the damage sugary drinks and foods do to people's teeth, yet nothing was said about sugar.

One of the speakers, Dr. Jane Kelly, the director of the National Diabetes Education Program for the Centers for Disease Control and Prevention, distributed literature that dentists could handout to their diabetic patients. While the handouts didn't blatantly encourage the consumption of sugar, there was no mention about restricting it either. Instead, the material recommended that diabetic patients should lose weight and eat less saturated fat and salt. In other words, eating sugar was fine as long as you maintain a healthy weight. But not all diabetics are overweight. To Kearns, the advice seemed ridiculous. It was like telling patients prone to tooth decay that they could eat all the sugar they wanted as long as they kept their weight under control.

In a handout from another keynote speaker, one of the recommended foods for diabetics was Lipton Brisk tea, a beverage containing the equivalent of 11 teaspoons of sugar per serving. As the speaker was leaving the conference, Kearns caught up to him and asked, "How can you say sweet tea is good for you?" He responded, "There is no research to support that sugar causes chronic disease." He then abruptly turned and left. Kearns was dumbfounded. How could leading health experts ignore the role of sugar in diabetes?

The lack of advice on sugar to diabetics at the conference seemed too conspicuous. Did science really support the omission, or were other forces at play? She wanted answers and began researching trade associations that promoted the consumption of sugar, looking for signs that they might be influencing the nutritional advice health-care workers give diabetics. She scoured the internet and pored over books at university libraries. After several months of searching, she found a library that had in its possession archived files from a bankrupt sugar company. In examining the files, she discovered confidential documents, internal memos, meeting minutes, and clues to other archives with more documents to be investigated. The documents clearly outlined the sugar industry's plot to influence medical research, government agencies, and public opinion. The involvement of the sugar industry was far greater than she could have ever imagined. It turned out that the "propaganda campaign," as it was sometimes referred to in the documents, succeeded in placing the blame of heart disease and other chronic illnesses on saturated fats, thus altering the course of nutritional science for the next 60 years.[15]

Internal memos revealed that early on the Sugar Association was aware of the links between sugar and chronic diseases. In 1954 they conducted a survey and found that the main reasons why customers limit sugar consumption at the time were:

1. It is fattening.
2. It causes cavities.
3. It causes diabetes.

An internal memo regarding this survey reads, "Therefore, in view of the above, the *propaganda campaign* just about to be started and continued for several years, will have to *destroy* these fallacies and at the same time *convince the people of the wholesome qualities* of sugar," (italics added).

The Sugar Association began funding studies to cast doubt on research that linked sugar consumption to various health problems. Researchers, such as Keys, Stare, and Hegsted were recruited to promote the fat hypothesis and downplay any involvement of sugar in the growing incidences of heart disease and diabetes. Vocal opponents, such as John Yudkin, were to be eviscerated and humiliated to discourage them and discredit their work.

The sugar industry worked to get sympathetic medical and research professionals into positions of authority in medical and government agencies. Throughout the 1960s, Keys secured places for himself and his allies on the boards of the most influential bodies in American healthcare, including the American Heart Association (AHA) and the National Institutes of Health (NIH). The Sugar Association managed to get other representatives appointed to positions of leadership and on advisory committees in the United States Department of Agriculture (USDA), the Centers for Disease Control and Prevention (CDC), and other influential organizations. From these positions of authority, they directed research funding to like-minded researchers, denied it to those unfriendly to the sugar industry, influenced federal policies, and issued nutritional advice to the nation.

The Sugar Association established a so-called independent scientific body consisting of physicians and dentists to defend sugar's place in a healthy diet. It was called the Food and Nutrition Advisory Council—a very scientific and impartial-sounding name that would give the organization the appearance of legitimacy and scientific authority. The newly formed Food and Nutrition Advisory Council wasted little time in compiling an 88-page booklet titled *Sugar in the Diet of Man*. The booklet's stated purpose was to organize existing scientific facts concerning sugar to dispel fears. The Sugar Association distributed 25,000 copies to the media and opinion makers. Accompanying the booklet was a news release with the headline "Scientists

Dispel Sugar Fears." Newspapers often reprint news releases word for word or with only minor editing as news stories.

From early on, the Sugar Association knew that if a product is perceived to be healthy, it will sell. So, they tried to transform sugar into a health food through the power of persuasive advertising. Although sugar has no redeeming health qualities, fictitious benefits were dreamed up and heavily promoted. It is well known that a lie repeated often enough is taken as the truth. The message was constantly repeated. Advertisements promoting sugar's assumed healthy image appeared everywhere in magazines, newspapers, and journals, and was broadcast on radio and television.

A headline on one 1954 advertisement reads: "What makes people fat?" The text follows: "People get fat simply because they overeat. Why do they overeat? Because they are hungry. Why are they hungry? One of the reasons in healthy individuals is because their blood sugar level is low. What is the fastest way to raise the blood sugar level and help keep from overeating? Sugar and the good things containing it!"

It continues: "Nutritional research has taken a new look at our number one health problem and discovered how sugar helps keep your appetite and weight under control."

The take-home message here is that we become fat by not eating enough sugar. Eat more sugar and you won't be hungry and overeat other foods. The text alludes to some unspecified "nutritional research" that is supposed to give these statements scientific legitimacy, so it must be true.

A 1959 ad headline reads: "Are you getting enough sugar to keep your weight down?" The text follows: "Sounds strange until you consider the necessity for appetite control when dieting. How do you curb a king-sized appetite? The easiest way is sugar. No other food satisfies your appetite so fast with so few calories. That's why you'll find sugar in so many modern reducing diets.

"Why today's active women need more sugar. You won't find the modern woman rocking on the porch. She's out bowling or golfing on weekends, and joining in the children's activities in between. This strenuous life requires energy—the kind sugar provides. That's why active people who know their energy needs include sugar in their diets."

This ad is written to appeal to the "modern" woman, who is more sophisticated and intelligent than her old-fashioned parents, who are too backward to appreciate the benefits of sugar. The older generation spends their time in rocking chairs because they have no energy—they don't eat enough sugar. Today's women are active and need the energy provided by sugar to accomplish everything they want to do.

The ad continues: "Sugar makes peaches taste peachier! All of us talk about tasting food, but now science tells us that your sense of smell is also

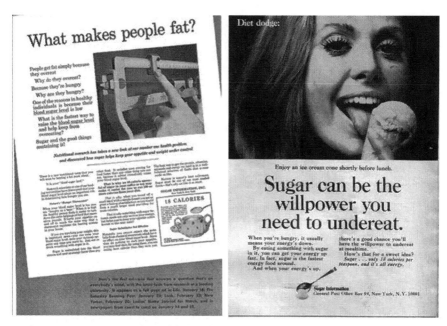

Advertising propaganda published by the sugar industry.

very important in your recognition of flavors. Recent experiments indicate that sugar releases hidden vapors in foods, delivers a stronger flavor message, helps you distinguish subtle differences."

There you have it. Science proves it: sugar is better. Simply adding sugar to foods brings out hidden vapors that activate smell receptors and enhance the taste of foods. May sound impressive, but where were these studies done and by whom? How do we know if these statements are true or they are just the imagination of some ad writer? Keep in mind that back in those days they didn't have all the laws we do now prohibiting false and misleading advertising, so an advertiser could say just about anything and get away with it, no matter how preposterous it may sound.

Believe it or not, a 1971 ad headline recommends, "An ice cream a day. . . Sugar can be the willpower you need to undereat." The ad continues: "When you're hungry, it usually means your energy's down. By eating something with sugar in it, you can get your energy up fast. In fact, sugar is the fastest energy food around. And when your energy's up, there's a good chance you'll have the willpower to undereat at mealtime. How's that for a sweet idea? Sugar . . . only 18 calories per teaspoon, and it's all energy."

If you have more energy, you will be able to resist overeating, so go ahead and enjoy that ice cream and you will eat less for dinner. I don't know about you, but eating ice cream never reduced my appetite. Sugar digests so quickly that an hour later the hunger is back.

Another 1970s ad headline reads: "If sugar is so fattening, why are so many kids so thin?" That ad wouldn't fly today. Obesity rates in adults and children have skyrocketed. By 2010, in the United States, 17 percent of kids ages 2-19 were obese.

On the podium of a Chicago ballroom in 1976, John Tatem Jr., the Sugar Association's president, and Jack O'Connell Jr., the association's director of public relations, were honored as the winners of the coveted Silver Anvil award. This prestigious honor is awarded by the public relations trade for excellence in "the forging of public opinion." Under the direction of these men, the Sugar Association pulled off one of the greatest coups in public relations history. For nearly a decade the sugar industry had withstood repeated criticism by scientists and the public, accusing sugar of causing obesity, diabetes, and heart disease, among other conditions. Ads claiming that sugar was an effective weight loss aid were questioned by the Federal Trade Commission (FTC) and the Food and Drug Administration (FDA), which launched a review of the evidence to see if sugar was even safe to eat. The Sugar Association's carefully crafted propaganda campaign successfully derailed the investigation and turned public opinion completely around to their favor. Association sponsored studies created doubt about sugar's negative reputation and shifted the blame to saturated fat. In the end, saturated fat was pegged as the villain and sugar was let off the hook.

In 1980, after much deliberation from a select group of America's most distinguished nutrition scientists, the US government issued its first *Dietary Guidelines for Americans*. The most prominent feature of the guidelines was the recommendation to cut back on the consumption of fat, saturated fats, and cholesterol. Avoiding excess consumption of sugar, primarily in the form of candy, was given as simply a means to reduce the risk of dental cavities and nothing more. Limiting sugar in other foods was not even mentioned. We were instructed to eat fish, poultry, and lean meat and to trim all excess fat off meats. We were told to limit the intake of all sources of saturated fat and cholesterol such as eggs, butter, cream, whole milk, coconut oil, and organ meats.

The government had given its official recommendations on a healthy diet based on the latest scientific evidence, so they had to be right. Doctors based their advice on these new guidelines; food companies developed products to comply with them. Low-fat diets became the rage. These guidelines shaped the diets of hundreds of millions of people not only in the United States but worldwide. In 1983, the UK government issued advice that closely resembled the American guidelines. Many other countries soon followed suit.

We dutifully complied with the dietary recommendations. We replaced steak and sausages with pasta and rice, butter with margarine and vegetable oils, eggs with cold breakfast cereals and pancakes, and whole milk with low-fat milk or orange juice. But instead of becoming thinner and healthier, we grew fatter and sicker. With the removal of saturated fat and cholesterol, we consumed more carbohydrate, primarily in the form of refined grains and sugars.

By 1999, Americans were consuming a record 152 pounds of added sweeteners each year, mainly in the form of sucrose and high-fructose corn syrup. This was 43 pounds more than was consumed during the 1950s. Needless to say, the official guidelines did not achieve their intended goal and actually led to a decades-long health disaster.

The War Goes On

Today the global sugar trade is worth $50 billion a year. The sugar industry pours millions into marketing and research to hide the truth and create confusion. They realize they can never win the debate about sugar's place in a healthy diet. Their primary argument is that there is no *conclusive* evidence linking sugar to chronic disease. At one time that may have been true, but not anymore. Evidence against sugar grows stronger every year. But the industry keeps fighting by funding studies to cause doubt and forestall or delay any scientific consensus against them.

In recent years, they appear to be grasping at anything to influence public opinion in their favor. One study, for example, claimed that candy consumption does not adversely affect health risk markers, and children in their study who ate candy bars were 22 percent less likely to be overweight.[16]

In 2015 the Coca-Cola Company, one of the members of the sugar industry's inner circle, rolled out a new campaign to promote the idea that it is not sugar that causes obesity but the lack of exercise. They founded a front organization by the name of Global Energy Balance Network, headed by university professors, to act as an impartial scientific committee to gather and conduct research supporting this concept and disseminate it to the media and the scientific community. The entire project was launched solely to create confusion in the minds of the public about the true cause of obesity and to steer blame away from sugar. However, by 2015 enough research had been published to refute the idea that obesity is caused primarily by the lack of exercise. The beverage company was caught red-handed. The deception received so much adverse publicity that Coca-Cola abandoned the idea.

The controversy continues and will probably do so for as long as the sugar industry continues its misinformation campaign, funding misleading studies and financially supporting scientists who promote the industry's agenda.

4

Sugar Isn't Always Sweet

CARBOHYDRATE IS SUGAR

We derive energy from the three macronutrients in our foods—carbohydrate, protein, and fat. While protein and fat can be used to produce energy, their primary function is to provide the basic building blocks for tissues, hormones, enzymes, and other structures that make up the human body. The primary purpose of carbohydrate, on the other hand, is to produce energy. It is the body's main source of fuel.

Carbohydrate is found in all plant foods. Milk is essentially the only animal-based food that contains any appreciable amount of carbohydrate. Plants are made predominantly of carbohydrate. Carbohydrates are constructed out of sugar. Sugar molecules provide the basic building blocks for all plants. The grass in your front yard, the flowers on your porch, the apples and oranges on your kitchen countertop, and the vegetables in your refrigerator are composed predominantly of sugar and water.

There are three basic types of sugar molecules that are important in our diet—glucose, fructose, and galactose. Essentially all the carbohydrates in our diet consist of some combination of these three. Simple carbohydrates consist of only one or two units of sugar. For example, table sugar, or sucrose, consists of one molecule of glucose and one of fructose. Milk sugar, or lactose, consists of one molecule of glucose and one of galactose. Complex carbohydrates are composed of many sugar molecules linked together by chemical bonds. Starch, for example, consists of long chains of glucose. Glucose is by far the most abundant sugar molecule in plant foods.

When you eat a slice of bread, you are eating mostly glucose in the form of starch. Along with the starch, you get some water, fiber (which is also a type of carbohydrate), vitamins, and minerals. The same thing is true when you eat an apple, a carrot, corn, potatoes, or any other plant-derived food.

When food containing carbohydrate is consumed, digestive enzymes break the bonds between the sugar molecules, releasing the individual glucose, fructose, and galactose molecules. These sugars are then transported to the bloodstream. Here glucose, also referred to as blood sugar, is delivered throughout the body to supply the fuel needed by the cells. Fructose and galactose, on the other hand, are taken up by the liver, converted into glucose, and then returned into the bloodstream. Foods high in glucose produce a rapid rise in blood sugar concentration. Fructose and galactose increase blood sugar as well, but not as rapidly, because they must pass through the liver first.

Dietary fiber is also a carbohydrate, but the human body does not produce the enzymes necessary to break the chemical bonds holding these sugars together. It passes through the body mostly intact until it reaches the last segment of the digestive tract, the colon, where the resident bacteria partially digest it and use it for their own nourishment. During this process the bacteria produce some vitamins and other nutrients that are absorbed and utilized by us. In this way, we form a symbiotic relationship with the bacteria where we both live together in a mutually beneficial way. We provide the bacteria a home and food, and they provide us with important nutrients. Since fiber releases little or no sugar, it does not raise blood sugar levels, nor does it have any of the detrimental effects associated with sugar.

The plants with the highest amount of carbohydrate are grains, legumes, and tubers (root vegetables, such as potatoes). These foods contain a high percentage of starch. Grains are of particular interest because in one form or another they constitute the vast majority of our diet. The grains we eat the most often have been refined—stripped of most of their fiber, fat, protein, vitamins, and minerals—leaving almost pure starch. These are referred to as refined carbohydrates. During digestion, starch is broken down into glucose. Most of the calories we get from starchy vegetables come from glucose.

Non-starchy vegetables, in contrast, don't provide much in the way of sugar calories. They consist mostly of water, generally comprising some 80 to 90 percent. The carbohydrate content is mostly in the form of fiber, which provides bulk to fill the stomach and satisfy hunger, but few calories. Foods rich in fiber are generally also rich in vitamins, minerals, and other important nutrients that support good health. Fruits have much of the same character and benefits as vegetables except they generally have a significantly higher sugar content.

With the exception of fiber, the carbohydrate in our food is eventually converted into a single form of sugar—glucose. This is the sugar that flows through our bloodstream. You often hear doctors speak of blood sugar or blood glucose. Glucose is important because it is the primary fuel that powers our cells and keeps us alive. In this respect, our bodies need sugar (glucose).

Since sugar is so important to our health, why is it considered harmful? It is not so much the sugar that is the problem; it is the overconsumption of sugar that causes trouble. It is much like alcohol in that you can consume a little without harm, but if you consume too much, it can cause a myriad of health problems; alcohol is also highly addictive and can easily lead to abuse. Likewise, sugar is generally harmless when consumed in moderation, but it is highly addictive, which can lead to sugar abuse and all of the health problems associated with it.

Simple sugars, such as sucrose, fructose, and glucose, are a greater problem than starch and complex carbohydrates rich in fiber. When consumed, sugars are immediately absorbed into the bloodstream, which can cause a great deal of stress on the body. Starch and other more complex carbohydrates, being composed of large chains of sugar, require a longer time to break down during the digestive process, releasing the sugars gradually into the bloodstream. Unless they are very refined, like white flour, they do not cause the stress that simple sugars do.

Simple Sugars
fructose
galactose
glucose
lactose (glucose + galactose)
sucrose (glucose + fructose)

SUGAR OVERLOAD

Companies put a great deal of effort into maximizing the allure of their products. One of the ingredients that greatly influences taste is sugar. Sugar, in one form or another, is found in the vast majority of commercially processed, packaged foods, whether they be sweet or savory.

The reason sugar is so pervasive in processed foods is due to the work of Howard Moskowitz, PhD, an American marketing researcher and psychophysicist. In the 1970s he was assigned the task of maximizing the appeal of Dr. Pepper. He tested 61 levels of sweetness to find the optimum level of sweetness to guarantee the new soda would fly off the shelf. This level is called the *bliss point*. It is the point at which the sweetness is the most desirable, sweet enough but not too sweet. The bliss point was first used in the formulation of soda, but is now used in all types of products—pasta sauce, cereals, tomato soup, bread, and so on. An unfortunate consequence of putting sugar in everything is that people tend to expect everything to have a slightly sweet taste. A generation of children has grown up eating foods sweetened to the bliss point. By comparison, real foods, such as vegetables, have become unappealing.

Sugar in foods, sweets, and snack foods has created a nation of sugar addicts. Sugar is so addictive that some people admit they can't live without it. They see a diet (low-carb, ketogenic) that eliminates all sugar and sweets and they claim such a diet is unrealistic and impossible to follow. How could it be impossible to follow? Most of the people who have lived on the earth throughout history followed a low- to no-sugar diet all their lives.

Keep in mind that sugar culture is a modern phenomenon. Our ancestors did not eat anywhere near the amount of sugar we do. They did not complain and did fine. They didn't feel they were suffering or deprived because they didn't have sugar every day (or for every meal). Sugar has been around for a long time. It was introduced into Europe nearly 1,000 years ago.

Before the 1960s sugar was only used occasionally, and generally only in desserts and sweets. Today it is consumed as a staple. Approximately 80 percent of the commercially prepared foods we eat contain added sugar.

Over the past 50 years, sugar consumption has tripled worldwide. Most of this is hidden sugar—sugar we don't realize we are eating. We may think we are eating a modest amount, but in reality we are consuming huge amounts even if we don't purposely add any sugar into our diets. The modern Western diet is loaded with hidden sources of sugar. Just because you don't add sugar to your foods or eat candy doesn't mean you are not consuming massive amounts of it. Sugar is obviously found in all sweetened foods, but it is also found as an ingredient in thousands of non-sweet products. You will find it in processed meats, bread and other baked goods, cereals, catsup and barbecue sauce, peanut butter, spaghetti sauce, canned goods, and frozen foods; it's even added to canned and frozen fruits and to most beverages. It's hard to find a packaged, prepared food that does not contain sugar or some other sweetener.

Today sugars come in a variety of forms, with names that are unfamiliar to many people. Here are just some of sugar's many names and varieties:

agave	fruit juice	molasses
barley malt	glucose	nonfat dry milk
brown rice syrup	high-fructose corn	palm sugar
brown sugar	syrup	saccharose
coconut sugar	honey	skimmed milk powder
corn syrup	lactose	sorghum
date sugar	levulose	sucrose
dextrin	maltodextrin	treacle
dextrose	maltose	turbinado
fructose	maple sugar	

Ingredient labels list the contents, starting with those that are the most predominant by weight, followed in order to the least. Sugar, with its various names, is often listed multiple times. In many packaged products, although sugar may not be listed first, if you combined all the many forms of sugar under the name "sugar," it often would become one of the first ingredients on the list.

The US Department of Agriculture (USDA) recommends that we limit our added sugar intake to no more than 6 percent of total daily calories or about 8 teaspoons (32 g) for an average-size adult. That would be far below the current level, and a sensible limit for most people.

The 8 teaspoons limit is for added sugars, the sugar you add to your coffee and cereal and use in your meal preparation, as well as the sugars manufacturers add to foods and beverages. This includes table sugar, corn syrup, high-fructose corn syrup, honey, and the like. It does not include the sugars found naturally in milk, fruit, and vegetables. Added sugar is always listed on the Nutrition Facts label so you can tell how much sugar a product contains.

Most people have no idea how much sugar they actually eat. One 12-ounce can of regular soda delivers 8 to 9 teaspoons of added sugar. Drinking just one soda puts you at or over your daily limit before you have eaten a single cookie or container of fruit-flavored yogurt or bowl of tomato soup or add a dressing to your salad. We get additional sugar that comes naturally in some foods. Fruits, and especially fruit juices, can be loaded with sugar, all of which contribute to your sugar overload.

So-called natural sugars, such as fruit juice concentrate or agave nectar, are no better than refined sucrose. The end results are the same. Whether you eat table sugar, honey, or molasses makes little difference.

SUCROSE

The sweetener we are all most familiar with and to which we compare other sweeteners is sucrose, or table sugar. This is the sugar commonly used in the home and in restaurants. It is the single most widely used sweetener in the home. Regardless of the source, most natural and refined sweeteners are primarily sucrose. Brown sugar, corn syrup, honey, and maple syrup are all primarily sucrose.

You will often hear that "natural" sweeteners are better than refined. The only advantage that natural sweeteners have is that they are less processed and therefore retain some of their nutritional value, but it isn't much. The most commonly used natural sweeteners are raw honey, unrefined maple syrup, dehydrated sugarcane juice, chopped dried dates, fruit juice concentrate, coconut sugar, and molasses. Like most sweeteners, these are made primarily of sucrose. Agave nectar or syrup, another product that is marketed as a natural sweetener, contains sucrose but is mostly fructose. Regardless of what you call them, the end results are the same. Sugar by any other name is still sugar.

Sucrose is composed of two other simpler sugars—glucose and fructose—each present in equal amounts. Each of these sugars has a distinct effect on our health. Let's take a look at each one.

GLUCOSE
Blood Sugar and Insulin Resistance

All digestible carbohydrate is eventually broken down and converted into glucose. As glucose circulates through the body, it is picked up by the cells and transformed into energy. The cells, however, cannot absorb glucose by themselves. They need the help of the hormone insulin. Insulin unlocks the door on the cell membrane, which makes it possible for glucose to enter. Without insulin, glucose cannot enter the cells. Your blood could be saturated with glucose, but if insulin was not present, glucose could not pass though the cell membrane.

Glucose is the primary source of fuel our cells use to produce energy. If the cells don't get enough glucose on a continual basis, they begin to degenerate and die. However, an overabundance of glucose is not good either. Too much glucose is toxic and can lead to mental confusion, coma, and death. To avoid the dire consequences of too little or too much glucose, the body has built in feedback mechanisms that maintain a narrow range of glucose levels in the blood.

Every time we eat, blood sugar levels rise. As sugar levels increase, special cells in the pancreas are triggered to release insulin into the bloodstream. As insulin shuttles glucose into the cells, blood sugar levels drop. At some point, another signal triggers the pancreas to stop insulin secretion. If blood sugar levels fall too low, the pancreas is prodded to release another hormone, called *glucagon*. Glucagon induces the release of glucose stored in the liver, thus increasing blood sugar levels. In this way, blood sugar is continually maintained within a narrow boundary.

Blood sugar levels naturally fluctuate slightly throughout the day. Whenever we eat, blood sugar levels increase. Between meals or during times of heavy physical activity, as the body's demand for energy increases, blood sugar levels decline. As long as the body is capable of compensating for both upward and downward spikes in blood sugar, balance is quickly reestablished and maintained.

What we eat profoundly affects the workings of this system. High-carbohydrate meals, especially if they contain a significant amount of simple carbohydrates and a lack of fiber, fat, and protein, can cause blood glucose levels to rise very rapidly. Refined starches, such as white flour, have been stripped of most of their fiber and bran and tend to act like sugar, spiking blood glucose levels as well.

Fiber, protein, and especially fat slow down the digestion and absorption of carbohydrate so glucose trickles gradually into the bloodstream, providing a steady, ongoing supply. The larger the quantity of simple and refined carbohydrate in meals, the greater the spike in blood sugar and the greater the strain placed on the body, and especially the pancreas, which produces both opposing hormones—insulin and glucagon.

If a high-carbohydrate meal is eaten every four or five hours, along with one or two high-carbohydrate snacks, such as a candy bar, soda, donut, or coffee with sugar between meals, insulin levels are going to be raised continually for a substantial part of the day. When cells are continually exposed to high insulin levels, they begin to lose their sensitivity to the hormone. It is like walking into a room with a bad odor. When you first enter the room, the smell can be overpowering, but if you have to stay in the room for any length of time, the smell receptors in your nose become desensitized and you will not notice the odor any longer. The smell is still there, but your ability to detect the smell has declined. If you left the room for a while and your sense of smell became resensitized, as soon as you walked back into the room you would again notice the odor. Our bodies react in somewhat the same way with insulin. Chronic exposure to high insulin levels desensitizes the cells, and they become unresponsive or resistant to the action of insulin. This is referred to as *insulin resistance*. In order to move glucose into the cells, a higher than normal concentration of insulin is needed, which puts more stress on the pancreas to produce more of the hormone. Insulin resistance is the hallmark feature and first step toward developing diabetes. It also takes you closer to obesity, heart disease, Alzheimer's, and many other degenerative diseases. Diet has a direct effect on the development of insulin resistance.

The two major forms of diabetes are designated as type 1 and type 2. Type 1 diabetes occurs when the pancreas is unable to produce a normal amount of insulin. This type of diabetes generally becomes evident in childhood or early adolescence and requires a lifetime of regular injections of insulin to keep blood sugar in balance.

In type 2 diabetes, the pancreas may be able to produce a normal amount of insulin, but the cells of the body have become unresponsive to the hormone. This is called insulin resistance. Over 90 percent of diabetics are of this type. Early in the course of the disease the pancreas is usually capable of producing the large amounts of insulin needed to overcome the insulin resistance of the cells. But over time the high demand for insulin takes its toll on the pancreas and insulin production begins to decline. Eventually the pancreas can burn itself out and stop producing the insulin needed. In this case, the diabetic needs supplemental insulin like a type 1 diabetic. More than half of all those with type 2 diabetes eventually require insulin to control their blood sugar levels as they get older. Type 2 diabetes is usually controlled with diet, weight management, exercise, and medication.

If you are an average, nondiabetic individual, when you wake up in the morning, your blood contains between 65 and 100 mg/dl (3.6-5.5 mmol/l) of glucose. This is known as the fasting blood glucose concentration. Fasting blood sugar measurements are taken after a person has not eaten for at least eight hours. The ideal fasting blood sugar range is between 65 and 90 mg/dl (3.6-5.0 mmol/l).

Diabetes is diagnosed when fasting blood sugar is 126 mg/dl (7.0 mmol/l) or higher. People with fasting blood sugar levels between 101 and 125 mg/dl (5.6-6.9 mmol/l) are considered to be in the early stages of diabetes, often referred to as *prediabetes*. Fasting blood sugar levels between 91 and 100 mg/dl (5.1-5.5 mmol/l) indicate the beginning stages of insulin resistance. As insulin resistance increases, so do blood sugar levels. The higher the blood sugar, the greater the insulin resistance.

The level at which a person is considered to have full-blown diabetes is defined as 126 mg/dl (7.0 mmol/l) or more, so does that mean if you have fasting blood sugar of 125 mg/dl (6.9 mmol/l) you are not diabetic and have nothing to fear? Not hardly. The 125 mg/dl (6.9 mmol/l) level indicates the presence of advanced insulin resistance that can lead to many serious health problems. Insulin resistance begins when fasting blood sugar levels rise over 90 mg/dl (5.0 mmol/l). Although levels up to 100 mg/dl (5.5 mmol/l) are generally considered normal, they are viewed this way only because so many people fit into this category. They are not really normal for a healthy individual. Having insulin resistance is not a state of health, even if the condition is relatively mild.

Diabetes was once a very rare condition. As sugar consumption has increased over the past century, the incidence of diabetes has also increased. At first, it seemed to only affect those populations that consumed modern processed foods loaded with sugar and refined flour. Over the past several decades, a tenfold increase in the incidence of type 2 diabetes has occurred worldwide. This has been documented in the Japanese, Israelis, Africans, Native Americans, Eskimos, Polynesians, Micronesians, and others.[1] This is believed to be caused by the increased availability and consumption of refined carbohydrates globally. Human population studies correspond with the animal studies that have clearly shown that diets very high in sugar are the underlying cause of insulin resistance and diabetes.

Some people are more susceptible to developing diabetes or insulin resistance than others. This susceptibility comes from their parents. Children of diabetic parents are at higher risk of developing insulin resistance and becoming diabetic themselves.[2]

If just one parent is insulin resistant, even if it is not severe enough to be diagnosed as full-fledged diabetes, the children can be at greater risk of developing insulin resistance. Mothers who develop gestational diabetes predispose their children to develop insulin resistance later in life. This is why diabetes sometimes seems to run in families. Susceptibility does not come from poor genes but from a poor diet. To make matters worse, poor eating habits are taught to children, who pass it down to their children. Consequently, people are developing diabetes at increasingly earlier ages.

In 1997, the United States government recommended that all adults be tested for diabetes by the time they reach age 45, before diabetic complications can progress and become difficult to treat. The rate of diabetes is increasing so fast that this recommendation is outdated. Today, the average age at which type 2 diabetes is diagnosed is 37. Researchers from the Centers for Disease Control and Prevention (CDC) are now recommending that people should be tested for type 2 diabetes at age 25.

Regardless of whether you are inherently susceptible to insulin resistance or diabetes, consuming high amounts of sugar and refined white flour greatly increases your risk. Eating a low-sugar or low-carb diet significantly reduces the risk.

The scientific evidence linking excess sugar consumption with increased risk of diabetes is strong.[3] A large analysis of worldwide sugar availability revealed that for every excess 150 calories of sugar (the amount in one can of soda), there was an eleven-fold increase in the prevalence of type 2 diabetes. No other type of food, including fat, yielded any significant association with diabetes. The duration and degree of sugar exposure correlated significantly with diabetes prevalence, while declines in sugar exposure correlated with significant subsequent declines in diabetes rates.[4]

Glycemic Index

It is primarily the glucose in sugar and other foods that has such a dramatic effect on blood sugar. Reducing the amount of glucose in our diet can have a significant impact on blood sugar levels. It's not always easy to tell which foods contain large amounts of glucose. In addition, some food components, such as fiber and fat, slow down the absorption of glucose into the bloodstream. For this reason, the glycemic index (GI) was developed. The glycemic index is a measure of how quickly certain foods raise blood sugar levels.

The GI is a scale from 0 to 100. Glucose is given the GI of 100, and all other foods are rated in comparison. The larger the number, the greater the effect a food has on blood sugar levels. Fiber, fat, and protein do not raise the GI, so foods rich in these nutrients are low on the scale. Foods rich in sugar or refined carbohydrate score high on the scale. For example, sucrose has a GI of 65, a banana has a GI of 51, and a slice of white bread 75. Note that white bread, although it may not taste as sweet as a banana, has a higher GI. The reason is that the banana also contains fiber that slows down sugar absorption. White bread, on the other hand, is mostly refined starch (glucose) with nearly all the fiber removed.

Chronic Inflammation

High glycemic index foods tend to increase systemic inflammation. When blood sugar levels rise, the sugar in your bloodstream tends to latch onto certain proteins in the blood vessel wall, causing injury and inflammation. When you eat high glycemic index foods repeatedly, your blood glucose levels are continually elevated, leading to chronic injury and inflammation. It is inflammation that causes cholesterol to become trapped in the artery wall. Without inflammation being present in the body, there is no way that cholesterol would accumulate in the wall of the blood vessel. Without inflammation, cholesterol would move freely throughout the body, as nature intended. This chronic inflammation of the arteries is one of the distinguishing features of atherosclerosis and coronary heart disease. In fact, chronic inflammation is associated with diabetes, obesity, Alzheimer's, cancer, and just about every other chronic degenerative disease.

Inflammation can be determined by measuring a marker in the blood called C-reactive protein (CRP); the higher the CRP, the more inflammation present. Your chance of developing any chronic disease increases progressively as CRP, or inflammation, increases. In the absence of an infection, a primary cause of inflammation is eating excessive amounts of sugar.[5-6] Sugar causes inflammation, eating sugar daily causes chronic inflammation, and chronic inflammation exponentially increases your chances of developing chronic disease.

Inflammation itself is another mechanism that damages the arteries and increases the risk of cardiovascular disease. Chronic inflammation injures tissues, causing the development of arterial plaque and atherosclerosis. While most other risk factors only indicate an association with heart disease,

61

arterial inflammation may be actively involved in its cause. The relationship between chronic arterial inflammation and heart disease is a much better indicator of heart disease risk than blood cholesterol levels.

Dr. Paul Ridker of Brigham and Women's Hospital in Boston evaluated blood samples from more than 28,000 healthy nurses. Those with the highest levels of C-reactive protein had more than four times the risk of having heart trouble. "We were able to find that the C-reactive protein is a stronger predictor of risk than were the regular cholesterol levels, and that's very important because almost half of all heart attacks occur among people who have normal cholesterol levels," he said.[7]

Inflammation of the arteries may explain heart disease in people without other known risk factors—people with normal cholesterol and low blood pressure who are nondiabetic and in good physical shape. These patients make up a third of all heart attack cases.

Advanced Glycation End Products (AGEs)

Sugar accelerates the aging process making you look and feel much older than you really are. Elevated blood glucose levels increase the rate of the formation of highly destructive molecular entities known as *advanced glycation end products* or AGEs. Glucose is a very sticky substance and combines easily with other molecules. In the bloodstream, if glucose is not quickly absorbed into the cells and used for the production of energy, it tends to stick or "glycate" with its surroundings. It can stick to fats but is especially attracted to proteins.

The effects of advanced glycation end products are aptly expressed in the acronym "AGE" because that's what they do—they age the body. Aging is the accumulation of damaged cells. The more AGEs you have in your body, the "older" you become functionally, regardless of how many years you've lived. AGEs adversely affect other molecules, generating free radicals, oxidizing LDL cholesterol (thus creating the type of cholesterol that collects in arteries and promotes atherosclerosis, heart attacks, and strokes), degrading collagen (the major supporting structure in our organs and skin), damaging nerve tissue (including the brain), and wreaking havoc on just about every organ in the body. AGEs are known to play an important role in the chronic complications of diabetes and in the development of Alzheimer's, Parkinson's, and other neurodegenerative diseases.[8-10]

The AGEs hypothesis of aging was prompted by multiple observations that aged tissues are characterized by the accumulation of a variety of AGE products. AGEs are involved in a vicious cycle of inflammation, generation of free radicals, amplified production of AGEs, more inflammation, and so on.

We all experience the effects of AGEs to some extent. It is just a part of living. As we grow older, we accumulate more AGEs and our bodies respond with the loss of elasticity and tone to skin and other tissues, decreased functional efficiency of organs, failing memory and motor skills, reduced ability to fight off infections, and all the other symptoms associated with aging.

Insulin resistance raises blood glucose levels. In diabetics glucose can remain abnormally high indefinitely, even with the use of medication. Chronically elevated blood glucose levels expose our cells and tissues to high concentrations of glucose for extended periods of time. The longer glucose is in contact with proteins, the greater the opportunity they have of forming advanced glycation end products. High blood sugar accelerates AGEing.

We are not totally defenseless against AGEs. They are so harmful that the body has a means of combating them. Our white blood cells have receptors specifically designed for them and latch onto the damaged proteins and remove them.

However, some glycated proteins, like those in collagen or nerve tissues, aren't easily removed. They tend to stick to each other and to other proteins, accumulating and causing damage to surrounding tissues. This plaque-like material becomes a more or less permanent fixture and a continual source of irritation. When a white blood cell encounters a glycated protein, it sets off an inflammatory reaction. The receptors for AGEs are known by the acronym RAGE, which is fitting since the reaction of white blood cells with AGEs can lead to chronic inflammation.

Diabetes is a major risk factor for heart disease. In fact, heart disease is the primary cause of death in diabetics. Heart disease is caused by diseased arteries. Studies have revealed that the destructive effect of AGEs on blood vessels accounts for the rapidly progressive atherosclerosis experienced by diabetics. It is this chronic high blood sugar characteristic of diabetes that leads to the deterioration of the arteries that causes peripheral vascular disease, diabetic retinopathy, kidney disease, and other diabetic complications.[11] For this reason, elevated blood sugar itself, whether diabetes is diagnosed or not, is considered a risk factor for heart disease.[12-14] Elevated blood sugar is referred to as *hyperglycemia.*

AGEs have been identified as the primary mechanism that initiates the steps that lead to the development of atherosclerosis. AGEs are highly damaging to the integrity and function of the blood vessel walls. They easily attach themselves to artery walls, generating free radicals and chronic inflammation. As tissues break down, proinflammatory cytokines, growth factors, and adhesion molecules are generated. Blood proteins, immune cells, LDL cholesterol, and fats infiltrate the damaged artery tissue where they are trapped. Cholesterol and fats are oxidized, and more inflammation is generated. Inflammation causes swelling of the artery, which constricts the artery canal, restricting blood flow and raising blood pressure. This leads to more injury to the artery wall, followed by more inflammation, scarring, and so forth. The process triggers a cycle of ongoing cellular injury and vascular dysfunction that characterizes atherosclerosis.[15] Blood levels of AGEs correlate well with the degree of atherosclerosis in both diabetics and nondiabetics with coronary heart disease.[16-17] Blood levels of AGEs have proven to be a useful predictor of coronary heart disease.[18]

According to the now outdated cholesterol hypothesis of heart disease, which many stubbornly refuse to abandon, it is the LDL cholesterol in the blood that for some unknown reason attaches itself to the artery wall, causing all the damage that leads to atherosclerosis and heart disease. However, cholesterol is a normal and natural product in our bodies; indeed, it is found in every cell and is essential for the proper function of our cells, not to mention its many other important purposes. If we don't get enough cholesterol in our diet, the liver makes it to satisfy our need for it. AGEs, on the other hand, serve no useful purpose. They are toxic by-products of nonenzymatic reactions between sugar and body tissues and are highly destructive.

AGEs tend to accumulate with age. However, higher levels seem to occur in certain disease states. In addition to diabetes and heart disease, elevated levels of AGEs are often associated with kidney disease, Alzheimer's disease, rheumatoid arthritis, and other maladies.[19] Research suggests that diets that raise blood sugar (e.g., diets high in sugar and refined carbohydrates), accelerate the consequences of natural aging and associated degenerative diseases.[20] One study reported that in a comparison of 172 young subjects (under 45 years of age) and older subjects (over 60 years), circulating AGEs increased with age. This was to be expected, but the researchers also found that indicators of inflammation, oxidative stress, and insulin resistance increased with AGEs regardless of the subject's chronological age.[21] AGE levels were more important in determining physical or functional age than was chronological age. It's not how old you are but how much accumulated damage you have sustained that really determines your level of health.

The formation of AGEs in our body is an ongoing process. While they can't be completely avoided, we can keep them to a minimum by reducing our sugar and refined carbohydrate consumption.

FRUCTOSE

If you read ingredient labels, you will frequently come across the words "fructose" or "high-fructose corn syrup." Fructose is found in all types of foods, from so-called health foods and dietary supplements to junk foods and candy. Fructose once gained a reputation as a "good" sugar primarily because it doesn't raise blood sugar and insulin levels the way sucrose does. For this reason, it has been the sugar of choice for many diabetics. Another reason for the popularity of fructose is that it is perceived to be more natural than sucrose and more healthful. It is often called "fruit" sugar, implying that its origin is from fruit rather than sugarcane or sugar beets and, therefore, is a less processed or more natural sweetener.

Unfortunately, this is just not so. Fructose is not, by any stretch of the imagination, a natural sugar, is not extracted from fruit, and is perhaps the most harmful sweetener a diabetic could use. The reason for much of this misinformation and its popularity is due to clever marketing tactics by the sugar industry.

High-fructose corn syrup was invented in 1957 by Richard Marshall and Earl Kooi, biochemists working for the Corn Products Company, a food ingredient company. Up until that time corn syrup was made entirely of glucose, containing no fructose. In their laboratory the researchers developed an enzyme called *glucose isomerase*, which could rearrange the molecular structure of glucose in corn syrup and convert it into fructose. Since fructose is sweeter than glucose, the more glucose that was converted into fructose, the sweeter the corn syrup became. This was a bonanza to the corn and sugar industries. Using high-fructose corn syrup in place of regular sugar, food products could be sweetened to the same degree of sweetness at less cost. High-fructose corn syrup began to be produced on an industrial scale in the early 1970s. Because of its low cost, high-fructose corn syrup quickly became the sweetener of choice in food manufacturing. Before 1970 most of the sugar we consumed was sucrose derived from sugarcane and sugar beets. In 1970 sucrose accounted for about 83 percent of the sweeteners consumed in America. By 1997 sucrose consumption had dropped to about 43 percent, with high-fructose corn syrup making up about 56 percent. Look at the ingredient labels of ice cream, candy, cookies, breads, and other prepared foods. If sugar is added, it most likely is in the form of high-fructose corn syrup.

The biggest myth about fructose is that it is fruit sugar and comes from fruit. The similarity between the words *fructose* and *fruit* helps perpetuate this myth. I've heard many a health food and supplement salesperson claim their product was superior to others because it was made with fruit sugar, meaning fructose.

Table sugar, or sucrose, is composed of equal amounts of glucose and fructose. High-fructose corn syrup in processed foods typically contains 55 percent fructose and 42 percent glucose, with the remaining 3 percent consisting of larger sugar molecules called *oligosaccharides*. While you get fructose from both sucrose and high-fructose corn syrup, there is one major difference. The fructose and glucose molecules in high-fructose corn syrup are free and unbound, ready for quick absorption. In contrast, every fructose molecule in sucrose is bound to a corresponding glucose molecule and must go through an extra metabolic step before it can be utilized. This rapid absorption of fructose and glucose from high-fructose corn syrup intensifies the detrimental effects of both.

Fructose has a much greater overall damaging effect on the body than glucose. We normally think of glucose when we talk about glycation, but fructose undergoes glycation at about 10 times the rate of glucose and intensifies AGE generation and tissue degeneration.

An interesting AGEs study was conducted in Europe. Researchers took two groups of nondiabetic subjects; one group was vegetarian and the other ate a mixed diet. Diet histories were recorded, and blood tests measured AGE levels. The results were surprising. You would expect that the vegetarians, who generally avoid fast food, eat more fruits and vegetables, and generally try to eat healthfully, would have lower AGE levels. But this was not the case. The mixed-diet subjects, who ate whatever they wanted, had significantly lower AGEs compared to the vegetarians. What was going on? The vegetarians ate two to three times as much fresh fruit as the mixed diet subjects, three times as much dried fruit, four times as much honey, and about the same amount of commercial sugar. The vegetarians' total sugar intake was significantly higher, particularly in fructose. The researchers attributed the higher AGE levels in the vegetarians to their high fructose consumption.[22] Even though their diet may have appeared to be healthy, their high sugar intake was setting the stage for premature aging and future health problems.

Nutritionists have been aware of the health problems associated with sucrose for some time. As questions about its safety emerged, researchers wanted to know whether it was the fructose or the glucose in the sucrose that was causing the most problems. The true nature of fructose was revealed by a team of USDA researchers led by Dr. Meira Field. They conducted studies with two groups of healthy rats, one given a diet with high amounts of glucose and the other with high amounts of fructose. Dr. Field found no obvious changes among the animals in the glucose group. However, in the fructose fed rats the results were disastrous. Young male rats were unable to survive to adulthood. They suffered from anemia, high cholesterol, and heart hypertrophy (their hearts enlarged until they ruptured). They also had delayed testicular development. Dr. Field explained that fructose in combination with copper deficiency in the growing animals interfered with collagen production. Collagen provides the protein matrix that holds our organs and tissues together. In humans, copper deficiency is common among those who eat a lot of processed convenience foods, as most people tend to do. The rats' bodies more or less just fell apart. The females were not as severely affected, but they were unable to produce live young.

"The medical profession thinks fructose is better for diabetics than sugar," says Dr. Field, "but every cell in the body can metabolize glucose. However, all fructose must be metabolized in the liver. The livers of the rats on the high fructose diet looked like the livers of alcoholics, plugged with fat and cirrhotic."[23]

When sucrose is consumed, the glucose and fructose molecules are split apart. The glucose goes directly into the bloodstream where it is used as fuel by the cells. Every cell in your body can metabolize glucose, but not fructose. Only the liver can metabolize fructose. Fructose goes directly to the liver where it is transformed into glucose and fat. In fact, fructose is more likely to be transformed into fat than into glucose. This is why fructose does not raise blood sugar levels as high as do sucrose or glucose. But it does raise blood triglyceride (fat) levels, more so than eating fat does. The high amount of fat produced from fructose metabolism clogs the liver, leading to fatty liver disease that resembles the damage caused by alcohol abuse. Doctors call it non-alcoholic fatty liver disease to distinguish it from the disease caused by excessive alcohol consumption. In addition to the excess fat, fructose causes liver cirrhosis and fibrosis.[24-25]

Cirrhosis of the liver develops when scar tissue replaces healthy tissue that has been damaged over a period of time, usually many years. Scar tissue makes the liver lumpy and hard and can lead to liver failure.

The detrimental effects of fructose on the liver are very similar to those of alcohol. See the similarities in the chart on the following page.

Fructose is far more fattening than other sugars or fat. Eating foods containing high-fructose corn syrup does not satisfy hunger but encourages overeating, which is another reason why food manufacturers prefer to use it in place of other sweeteners. Fructose tricks you into gaining weight by turning off your body's appetite control system. Fructose does not appropriately stimulate insulin, which in turn, does not suppress ghrelin, the hormone that stimulates hunger, and does not activate leptin, the hormone that suppress hunger. This leads to overeating and weight gain.

Fructose not only stimulates overeating, but it is preferentially converted into fat in comparison to glucose. Researchers at Princeton University found that when rats were given access to high-fructose corn syrup, they gained significantly more weight (stored more fat) than those with access to sucrose, even when their overall caloric intake was the same.[26] In addition to causing significant weight gain, long-term consumption of high-fructose corn syrup leads to abnormal distribution of body fat, preferentially

Liver Toxicity

Excessive consumption of fructose can cause many symptoms similar to alcohol abuse.

Chronic Ethanol Consumption	Chronic Fructose Consumption
Haematological disorders	-
Electrolyte abnormalities	-
Hypertension	Hypertension (uric acid)
Cardiac dilatation	-
Cardiomyopathy	Myocardial infarction (dyslipidaemia, insulin resistance)
Dyslipidaemia	Dyslipidaemia (*de novo* lipogenesis)
Pancreatitis	Pancreatitis (hypertriglyceridaemia)
Obesity (insulin resistance)	Obesity (insulin resistance)
Malnutrition	Malnutrition (obesity)
Hepatic dysfunction (alcoholic steatohepatitis)	Hepatic dysfunction (non-alcoholic steatohepatitis)
Fetal alcohol syndrome	-
Addiction	Habituation, if not addiction

Source: Lustig, RH, et al. The toxic truth about sugar. *Nature* 2012;482:27-29.

collecting in the abdominal area, causing a big belly. Belly fat is known as visceral fat. This is the fat that is stored within the abdominal cavity; it is not the same as the fat that collects under your skin, but accumulates around your organs—around your liver, heart, and intestines. It causes the belly or waistline to bulge out. Visceral fat is not just excess fatty tissue, but metabolically active tissue that releases hormones and promotes inflammation and increases your risk of a number of health problems, including obesity, heart disease, diabetes, cancer, depression, arthritis, sexual dysfunction, sleep disorders, and dementia.

"Some people have claimed that high-fructose corn syrup is no different than other sweeteners when it comes to weight gain and obesity, but our results make it clear that this just isn't true," says Dr. Bart Hoebel, who specializes in the neuroscience of appetite, weight, and sugar addiction at Princeton. "When rats are drinking high-fructose corn syrup at levels well below those in soda pop, they're becoming obese—every single one, across the board. Even when rats are fed a high-fat diet, you don't see this: they don't all gain extra weight."[27]

In the Princeton study the concentration of sugar in the *sucrose solution* was the same as that found in most soft drinks. However, the *fructose solution* was only half as concentrated as most sodas but still produced far greater weight gain and body fat accumulation in comparison.

In long-term studies lasting over 6 months, the animals eating a diet with added fructose showed signs of a dangerous condition know in humans as *metabolic syndrome*, which greatly increases the risk of obesity, heart disease, diabetes, and many other degenerative conditions. In one study, it was found that male rats, in particular, ballooned in size; animals with access to fructose gained 48 percent more weight than those eating a normal diet. Putting this into human terms, a 200-pound person would put on an additional 96 pounds! The rats weren't just growing fat; they were becoming obese.

High-fructose corn syrup is found in a wide range of foods and beverages, including fruit juice, soda, cereal, bread, yogurt, ketchup, mayonnaise, and salad dressings. On average, Americans consume 60 pounds of the sweetener per person every year. In the 40 years since the introduction of high-fructose corn syrup as a cheap sweetener in the American diet, rates of obesity in the United States have skyrocketed, according to the Centers for Disease Control and Prevention (CDC). In 1970, about 15 percent of the US population met the definition for obesity; today, over 30 percent of the American adults are considered obese, and 3 out of 4 are overweight.

Another problem with fructose is that while it does not immediately affect blood sugar and insulin levels as much as glucose, it has a more detrimental effect on insulin resistance, increasing the risk of a number of health problems like heart disease, high blood pressure, and diabetes. Studies on both animals and humans have shown that consuming large amounts of fructose impairs the body's ability to properly handle blood glucose, which ultimately leads to elevated glucose levels and the development of insulin resistance. This fact is so well established now that researchers use fructose to intentionally induce insulin resistance, create high blood pressure, and initiate diabetes in laboratory animals. Some physicians are now claiming that the increased use of fructose in all our foods is largely responsible for the skyrocketing incidence of diabetes we are experiencing today.

Fructose has also been shown to increase the rate at which fats in our body undergo peroxidation, which produces destructive free radicals. It adversely affects blood lipids and blood pressure, increasing risk of cardio-vascular disease, and interferes with nutrient absorption.[28]

Fructose is everywhere. You get it from commercial food products and from the sugar you use at home. Remember that table sugar is 50 percent fructose. All sources of fructose have the same effect on the body. It does not matter if the fructose is from high-fructose corn syrup, sucrose, or a natural source, such as agave syrup (a popular sweetener used in the health food industry). The effects are all the same.

Agave syrup is often marketed as a healthy alternative to table sugar or high-fructose corn syrup because it does not spike blood sugar as sucrose does. However, the reason it doesn't is because it is made predominantly of fructose.

Agave marketers portray their product as a natural sweetener straight from the sap of the agave plant and advertise it as "diabetic friendly," "raw," and "100% natural." Nothing could be further from the truth. Agave nectar, as it is sometimes called, generally does not come from the sap but from starch derived from the root. The enzymatic process is similar to that of turning cornstarch into high-fructose corn syrup. It is nothing more than a commercially produced, super-condensed form of fructose syrup. High-fructose corn syrup has a fructose content of 55 percent, the fructose content of agave syrup ranges up to 70 to 97 percent, depending on the brand. Despite the misinformation from marketers, agave syrup or nectar is far worse for your health than any other form of sugar.

GALACTOSE

Milk sugar, or lactose, consists of equal amounts of glucose and galactose. In some respects galactose is similar to fructose. Like fructose, it must be converted into glucose by the liver before being released into the bloodstream, putting excess stress on the liver and promoting fat synthesis and the increase of blood triglyceride levels. And like fructose, it is 10 times more susceptible to forming AGEs than glucose. Unlike fructose, galactose isn't very sweet; it is only 35 percent as sweet as sucrose and less than half as sweet as glucose.

The consumption of typical quantities of whole milk, cream, cheese, and other natural dairy products does not expose us to any appreciable amount of galactose that would be of concern. However, when fat is removed from whole milk to make nonfat and low-fat milks, yogurt, and other dairy products, the percent of sugar in the remaining milk significantly increases. This type of sugar occurs naturally, so it is not listed on food labels.

Nonfat dried milk is used in many low-fat dairy products to make up for the loss of flavor from the removal of the fat. Whenever you see nonfat dried milk added to a food, you should consider it as if it were high-fructose corn syrup, as the consequences are similar. Many people would avoid buying cottage cheese, yogurt, or cream if high-fructose corn syrup were added, but not give it a second thought if it contained nonfat dried milk. Nonfat dried milk is often added to reduced-fat milks to give them more body and flavor. All reduced-fat milk and milk powders are potential sources of excessive amounts of galactose.

Nonfat dry milk and skimmed milk powder are used in many processed foods. Both are very similar, the primary difference is that skimmed milk powder has a minimum milk protein content of 34 percent, whereas nonfat dry milk has no standardized protein level. According to the US Dairy Export Council, both powders typically consist of between 49.5 and 52 percent lactose.[29] In other words, nonfat dry milk is about 25 percent galactose and 25 percent glucose, which means that nonfat dry milk is predominantly sugar.

Like fructose, galactose is well known for promoting premature aging, inflammation, and excessive oxidative stress and vitamin deficiencies due to the production of AGEs and free radicals. The consumption of high levels of galactose rapidly age the body and the cardiovascular system, increasing the risk of heart attack and stroke. Since 1991 galactose has been used in animal research to explore the effects of aging on the heart.[30]

While some researchers recognize that galactose can induce premature aging on the heart and increase the risk of heart disease, others have ignored these findings in their zeal to link milk fat or cholesterol to cardiovascular disease. A number of studies have evaluated the effects of dairy consumption on cardiovascular disease risk, focusing primarily on the fat content, while ignoring other components, such as lactose and galactose. In general, the results have been mixed, with no clear indication that saturated fat or cholesterol in the dairy increase heart disease risk.

William B. Grant, PhD, at NASA Langley Research Center in Hampton, Virginia, has noted that the mixed results are due to the fact that milk sugar and nonfat milk are higher risk factors for heart disease than either cholesterol or saturated fat, neither of which was controlled for in these studies.[31]

Grant used data from 32 countries to look for links between heart disease and dairy consumption. Milk carbohydrates were found to have the highest statistical association with ischemic heart disease for males aged 35 and older and for females aged 65 and older. For females ages 35-64, sugar was found to have the highest association. In the case of coronary heart disease, nonfat milk was found to have the highest association for males aged 45 and older and females aged 75 and older, while for females 65-74, milk carbohydrates and sugar had the highest associations, and for females aged 45-64, sugar had the highest association.[32]

A recent study published in the *British Medical Journal* indicated that drinking milk, and especially nonfat milk, might increase a person's risk of dying from heart disease and suffering bone fractures. The study examined dietary habits of more than 100,000 people living in Sweden. The study tracked 60,000 women for 20 years and 45,000 men for 11 years. Those who drank more than 3 glasses (about 3 cups or 680 ml) of milk per day were more likely to die over the course of the study and to suffer a bone fracture. The effect was most pronounced among women, who were nearly twice as likely to die from heart disease—the condition with the strongest links to the high milk consumption.[33]

The researchers did not make a distinction between whole, nonfat, or low-fat milk but did note that heart disease risk as well as bone fractures actually decreased with the consumption of fermented milk (yogurt/kefir) and cheese. Since most people are fearful of saturated fat and weight conscious, they tend to prefer drinking reduced-fat milks. The researchers speculated that the reason for the high cardiovascular risk was probably due to the galactose content of the subjects' diet. In this study, milk consumption was positively associated with increased oxidative stress and inflammation, both of which are known responses to galactose consumption. Fermented milks and cheese, which have lower galactose levels, were not associated with oxidative stress or inflammation.

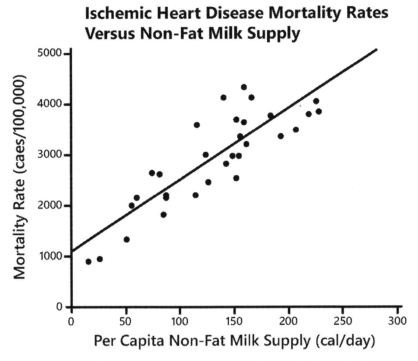

Ischemic heart disease mortality rates, males aged 75 and older versus nonfat milk supply available in 32 countries, 1983. Source: Grant, WB. Milk and other dietary influences on coronary heart disease. Altern Med Rev1998;3:281-294.

There have been many populations around the world that rely heavily on dairy as their primary source of food. Classic examples include the residents of the Lötschental, a valley in Switzerland, and the Maasai in East Africa. The Lötschental valley, which is surrounded by three snowcapped mountain ranges, has been mostly isolated from the rest of the country. For generations the people had to rely on locally produced food, the majority of which consisted of dairy. When Weston A. Price visited the area in the 1930s, he found the people to be in excellent health. There was no evidence of heart disease, cancer, tuberculosis, or other diseases that were common in Europe and America. The residents' dental health was also exceptional, even in the absence of dentists and with total disregard for regular dental hygiene.

The Maasai are a pastoral people inhabiting Kenya and northern Tanzania. Traditionally, the Maasai were seminomadic and their diet consisted almost entirely of milk from their cattle, supplemented occasionally with blood and meat. Each person would consume several quarts of milk daily. The Maasai were famed for their physical strength and bravery and were considered fierce warriors. Despite their high milk and saturated fat consumption, they have been completely immune to cardiovascular disease, diabetes, cancer, and other degenerative diseases until more recent times, as they have adapted to agriculture and a diet much higher in carbohydrate-rich foods.

Consuming large quantities of whole milk and cream have never been a problem for those people throughout history who have used dairy products liberally. Even the consumption of several quarts of whole milk daily has not had a detrimental effect. In fact, dairy consumption has always been considered to be healthful. However, the use of nonfat milk and milk powders has greatly increased galactose intake, which apparently nullifies the many health benefits that come from dairy consumption, such as protection from heart disease and bone fractures, and increases the effects of aging.

Like high-fructose corn syrup, galactose in the form of nonfat milk and milk powders, is now used in a multitude of processed food products. It is found in most all low-fat dairy products, including cottage cheese, cheese, cheese spread, yogurt, and ice cream, as well as milk chocolate, dessert and pudding mixes, chocolate milk mix, gravy mix, cookie dough, and processed lunch meats. It is also a popular ingredient in many dry goods, such as pancake and biscuit mixes, cake mix, cookies, crackers, bread, and other bakery and confectionery products. If that isn't bad enough, you can buy pure nonfat dry milk to make your own reconstituted nonfat milk.

In addition to the sugar, dried milk also contains up to 30 mcg/g of oxidized cholesterol.[34] Undamaged cholesterol is not harmful and is actually beneficial. It is only the damaged or oxidized cholesterol that is harmful to the arteries and can cause damage that promotes atherosclerosis.[35] Dried whole milk powder contains more oxidized cholesterol and fat than nonfat dried milk, making it potentially just as harmful.

5

A Weapon of Mass Destruction

SUGAR'S EFFECT ON HEALTH

According to the World Health Organization (WHO) noncommunicable, or chronic, diseases kill 41 million people each year, equivalent to 71 percent of all deaths globally.[1] The vast majority of these deaths, some 80 to 90 percent, is diet related and includes cardiovascular diseases, diabetes, obesity, and cancer. The incidence of these diseases has risen sharply over the past few decades as dietary patterns have changed and manufactured, processed foods have displaced traditionally prepared foods. The biggest change in the diet has been the addition of sugar. We consume more sugar now than at any time in history, much of it in the form of sugary drinks, which are now available in even the remotest parts of the world. In areas where the water is often unsafe to drink unless treated, the people rely heavily on colas and other sugary beverages. The consequences have been devastating, leading to an epidemic in diabetes and heart disease. The introduction of sugar and sugary drinks has been a curse, causing death and disabilities in areas where just a few decades earlier such diseases were rare or unheard of. The spread of sugar-filled junk foods worldwide has led to more deaths and disabilities than any plague or war in history. Sugar can truly be considered a weapon of mass destruction.

The health threat from the overconsumption of sugar is real, and it doesn't take much added sugar to have a significant impact. To put it bluntly, sugar kills—slowly, but it kills. It kills by accelerating the rate of aging and degeneration, leading to chronic diseases that cause disability and death.

Many government and international health organizations have issued reports warning about the dangers of consuming too much sugar. Based on the published research, these reports conclude that a high intake of added sugar increases the risk of obesity, type 2 diabetes, high blood pressure, stroke, heart attack, senility, mental illness, liver disease, kidney disease, cancer, gallstones, arthritis, and dental cavities. The list of problems can go on and on.

In addition, foods with added sugar are generally low in essential nutrients and fiber. Consuming such food displaces more nutrient-dense foods, leading to weight gain and malnutrition. To make matters worse, sugar has proven to be highly addictive, like tobacco and alcohol, compelling us to consume it and overconsume it, despite our better judgment and efforts at self-control. When you look at all the evidence, most of the major chronic health problems we face today are directly related to sugar consumption, not to fat.

In this chapter we will examine some of the major documented problems associated with our love affair with sugar.

UNHEALTHY DIET

An unhealthy diet is the root cause of many chronic and degenerative diseases. It is a recognized risk factor for heart disease. The term "unhealthy diet" is another way of saying a high-sugar diet without saying the word "sugar." This keeps the sugar industry happy. This classification is ambiguous because everybody has their own definition of a "healthy" diet. However, most everyone will agree that any diet that is low in nutrition and high in empty calories is an unhealthy diet. Sugar, refined grains, and overly processed high-carb fruits and vegetables, such as fruit leather and potato chips, fit the definition of foods that supply empty calories with little nutrition. On the contrary, fresh fruits, vegetables, nuts, whole grains, dairy, eggs, and meats all supply a rich variety of essential nutrients and would not be classified as empty-calorie foods.

The overconsumption of sugar at the expense of healthier foods leads to an unhealthy diet lacking in essential vitamins, minerals, antioxidants, fiber, and other essential nutrients that leaves the body malnourished and open to premature aging and degenerative disease.

Sugar Addiction

Our love affair with sweets has created a society of sugarholics. Sugar is dangerously addicting, much like narcotics. Like cocaine and other drugs, they stimulate pleasure centers in the brain. The desire for this pleasurable sensation can become so intense that it controls our thoughts and actions, just as cocaine controls an addict.

Sweets have never been a major source of food in the human diet. In the past, fruit provided the majority of our sweets. Since fruit was only available during the summer, it was only eaten a few months out of the year. The lack of refrigeration prevented the storage of fruits for long periods of time. While refined sugar has been around for a few hundred years, it never was a major part of the diet.

Addiction involves more than just a preference for something because you like the taste. It can be defined as the persistent compulsive use of a substance that on cessation causes psychological or physical anxiety. Sugar cravings fit into this definition. Sugar can be just as addictive, and even more so, than cocaine. This may sound like an overstatement because a person can stop eating sugar without suffering from the severe physical withdrawal symptoms commonly associated with cocaine addiction. Nevertheless, sugar addiction can cause dependence, severe anxiety, and even physical symptoms upon withdrawal.

A study published by French researchers demonstrated just how addicting sugar can be. Given the choice between sugar or cocaine, they found that 94 percent of rats chose sugar. When exposed to both substances, their desire for sugar was stronger than the desire for cocaine. Even rats who were already addicted to cocaine quickly switched their preference to sugar as soon as they were offered the choice. The rats were also more willing to work for sugar than for cocaine.[2]

In addition, the researchers found that there is a cross-tolerance and a cross-dependence between sugar and addictive drugs. As an example, animals with a long history of sugar consumption actually became tolerant (desensitized) to the analgesic effects of morphine.

A study out of Yale University found that addictions to sugar and drugs result in similar activity in the brain. Test subjects filled out a questionnaire, based on established criteria for accessing drug addiction, to measure their addiction to certain foods. The questionnaire included statements such as, "I find that when I start eating certain foods, I end up eating much more than I had planned," and respondents rated how closely the statements matched their experiences.

Using magnetic resonance imaging (MRI), a brain imaging procedure, the researchers examined brain activity when the subjects saw, and then drank, a chocolate milkshake. What they found was that the brains of subjects who scored higher on the food addiction scale exhibited brain activity similar to that seen in drug addicts, with greater activity in brain regions responsible for cravings and less activity in the regions that curb urges.[3]

As with drug addiction, cutting down on sugar and carbohydrate consumption all at once can cause withdrawal symptoms. Symptoms may include intense carbohydrate cravings, headache, lightheadedness, irritability, irrational behavior, fuzzy thinking, and a overall feeling of tension or stress.

Low-calorie sweeteners do not help with overcoming sugar addiction. They give you a false sense of security while fueling the fire of sugar addiction. Studies that showed sugar to be more addictive than cocaine also showed zero-calorie sweeteners were just as addictive. Using sugar substitutes keeps sugar addictions, cravings, and bad habits alive.

One of the big problems with both sugar and artificial sweeteners is that because they stimulate pleasure centers in our brain, we tend to overeat. Most sweetened foods are high in calories and low in nutrition. Therefore, we tend to fill up on nutritionally deficient, calorie-rich, artificially flavored foods, leaving little room for nutritionally dense, high-fiber, wholesome foods. When children grow up eating nutritionally poor foods, these are the foods they learn to like. Consequently, as they become adults they continue to eat these types of foods, and suffer the consequences of poor health and obesity as a result.

Like a drug addict, who needs a larger and larger dose to achieve the same effect, we need more and more sugar in our foods to enjoy the same level of sweetness or get the same amount of pleasure.

With sugar addiction, we tend to prefer foods that are sweetened, even those foods that normally have little or no sugar like meats and vegetables. After a while, natural foods that are unsweetened gradually become less appealing. This is one reason why sugar is often added to frozen fruit and why canned fruits are packed in syrup. Fresh fruit just isn't sweet enough anymore.

Desensitizing taste receptors makes ordinary vegetables and other natural foods less appealing. Kids nowadays don't like vegetables. In our great-grandparents' day kids ate their vegetables; they didn't turn up their noses at peas and broccoli as they do now. Nor did they get soda pop, candy, and sugar coated breakfast cereal every day. Kids don't like vegetables because their taste buds are desensitized from eating too much sugar and artificial sweeteners. Many adults don't care much for vegetables for the same reason. If fresh, unsweetened fruits and vegetables aren't appealing to you, you're not going to eat them. Instead, you wind up eating less healthy foods, which keep your sweet cravings alive.

Rats given a choice will consume sugar water in preference to a nutritious diet, even to the point of malnutrition and death. We seem to be doing the same, consuming sugary foods to the point of malnutrition, which ultimately leads to chronic disease and death.

Subclinical Malnutrition

A study published in *BMJ Open* found that nearly 60 percent of foods eaten in America are ultra-processed, convenience foods. *Ultra-processed* as defined by the study are those foods that include multiple ingredients and additives, such as flavorings, colorings, sweeteners, emulsifiers, and such. Most boxed, canned, packaged, and ready-to-eat frozen foods fit into this category. The researchers also found that on average, 20 percent of the calories in ultra-processed foods come from sugar and that these foods account for nearly 90 percent of the added sugar in the US diet.[4-5]

This situation isn't unique to the United States. Most Westernized countries have similar eating patterns.

As sugar-laden processed food consumption has increased over the years, more nutritious foods have been pushed out. Instead of eating fresh fruits, vegetables, and whole grains, we eat white bread, chips, crackers, sugary breakfast cereals, and all manner of sweetened and refined carbohydrate-rich foods. Other than the calories it supplies, sugar provides no nutritional value. It contains no vitamins, minerals, or other nutrients. It is a source of empty calories.

Taking a multivitamin supplement or adding vitamins to fortify an otherwise nutritionally depleted breakfast cereal doesn't make it any healthier. High sugar intake contributes to nutrient deficiencies in ways other than by just displacing more nutritious foods. Sugar actually depletes or reduces the absorption of certain vitamins and minerals. As a result, eating too much sugar can induce deficiencies, even when the overall nutrient intake appears to be adequate. It is, in fact, an antinutrient. It robs the body of nutrients vital to good health. The consumption of sugar causes the body to use up its supplies of calcium, magnesium, potassium, thiamine, and chromium in the process of metabolizing the sugar. Sugar robs the body of vitamin C by competing with it for transportation into cells. Overconsumption of sugar can cause a vitamin C deficiency, leading to subclinical scurvy. A disease that is subclinical means the condition is present but not yet advanced enough to be detectable through conventional diagnostic methods.

If you eat more than 200 grams of carbohydrate in a day (300 grams is common), mostly from refined grains and sugar, and do not eat much fresh fruit or vegetables, You are most likely vitamin C deficient, even if you are consuming the recommended dietary allowance (RDA) of vitamin C (in the United States it is 60 mg/day). If you are diabetic or prediabetic, the risk of deficiency is even greater.

Glucose and vitamin C molecules are very similar in structure. Most animals can make their own vitamin C from glucose derived from the carbohydrates in their diets. It is a very simple process. Humans, however, cannot. We do not have the enzymes that can make this conversion, so we must get our vitamin C directly from the foods we eat. The similarity between glucose and vitamin C extends beyond the molecular structure but also includes the way they are attracted to, and enter, cells. Both molecules require help from insulin before they can penetrate cell membranes.

Glucose and vitamin C compete with each other for entry into our cells. But this competition is not equal. Our bodies favor glucose entry at the expense of vitamin C. When blood glucose levels are elevated, vitamin C absorption into the cells is severely restricted. Whenever you eat a meal that contains carbohydrate, it will be converted into glucose, which will interfere with vitamin C absorption. The more carbohydrate you eat, the higher your blood glucose goes, and the less vitamin C your body utilizes. It is ironic that you can drink sweetened orange juice or sugary breakfast cereals that are fortified with extra vitamin C, yet the sugar in these products almost completely blocks the absorption of the vitamin. A high-sugar diet can lead to vitamin C deficiency. If a person is diabetic or is insulin resistant (even a little), blood glucose is elevated for extended periods of time, blocking vitamin C absorption even more.

For this reason, diets high in sugar and refined starch can cause vitamin C deficiency. The effect of sugar on blocking the absorption of vitamin C is highly significant, yet generally unrecognized by the medical profession. It is possible to develop severe vitamin deficiency even when the diet contains what we might consider ample sources of vitamin C.

A study published in the *International Journal of Vitamin Research* found that vitamin C status can improve significantly simply by removing sugar and refined starch from the diet.[6] The more sugar you eat, the greater your vitamin C levels decline. When a diet is loaded in sugar and refined starch, vitamin C deficiency can lead to subclinical scurvy.

Scurvy results from severe vitamin C deficiency. Symptoms include anemia, depression, frequent infections, bleeding gums, loosened teeth, muscle degeneration and pain, joint pain, slow healing of wounds and injuries, and the development of atherosclerosis. Atherosclerosis leads to heart attacks and strokes. It is far more likely for you to suffer a heart attack or stroke from eating a vitamin C–robbing, high-sugar diet than by eating a high-fat diet.

Vitamin C is just one of the many essential nutrients that is deficient in a diet overloaded with sugar-laden processed foods. The US Department of Agriculture states that most of us don't get enough (100 percent RDA) of at least 10 essential nutrients. Only 12 percent of the population obtains 100 percent of seven essential nutrients. Less than 10 percent of us get the recommended daily servings of fruit and vegetables. Forty percent of us eat no fruit and 20 percent no vegetables. And most of the vegetables we do get are fried potatoes—a rich source of starch.

When we think of malnutrition, we usually think of emaciated drought victims in Africa or starving people in India. In more affluent countries, the problem is more insidious. Symptoms of malnutrition are not as evident. People don't look malnourished, and methods of diagnosing deficiency diseases require malnutrition to be in a more advanced stage before they can be detected.

When a variety of foods are available, few people develop obvious symptoms of malnutrition, even when their diets are nutritionally poor. Instead, they suffer from subclinical malnutrition. This condition can go on unnoticed indefinitely. In Western countries subclinical malnutrition is epidemic. Our foods are sadly depleted of nutrients. We eat and eat and even overeat to the point of becoming overweight yet still are malnourished. As a result, the immune system is chronically depressed, the body cannot fight off infections well, and tissues and cells starving for nutrients slowly degenerate and all manner of chronic disease creeps in.

Homocysteine

In recent years, elevated blood levels of homocysteine (a sulfur-containing amino acid) has gained recognition as an important risk factor for heart disease. It has been linked to increased risk of heart disease and stroke even among people who have normal cholesterol levels. Elevated homocysteine levels appear to damage cells lining the inside of the arteries, leading to atherosclerosis. Studies indicate that elevated blood homocysteine levels are more accurate in predicting heart disease than high cholesterol, high blood pressure, or cigarette smoking. A review of all published studies on homocysteine indicates that it is one of the most significant, independent risk factors for atherosclerosis. For every 10 percent elevation of homocysteine, there is a corresponding rise in the risk of developing severe coronary heart disease.[7]

The connection between homocysteine and cardiovascular disease was first suspected about 40 years ago when it was observed that people with a rare genetic condition called *homocystinuria* (elevated homocysteine levels) were prone to develop severe cardiovascular disease. One of the first reported cases involved an 8-year-old who exhibited all the signs of advanced atherosclerotic disease and died of a stroke—a curious death for someone so young. Atherosclerosis and stroke are considered diseases of aging.

Homocysteine is derived from the metabolic breakdown of methionine—one of the essential amino acids obtained from dietary protein in our food. Methionine is more common in animal proteins than in vegetable proteins. When we eat protein-rich foods, methionine is converted into homocysteine. The liver converts homocysteine back into methionine or into other substances, so the concentration is normally very low. Too much homocysteine is toxic to the arteries and can both initiate and accelerate atherosclerosis.

Dangerously elevated homocysteine levels can occur in anyone as a result of an improper diet. The enzymes that metabolize homocysteine and convert it back to methionine are dependent on three B vitamins: B_6, B_{12}, and folic acid. Abnormal elevation of homocysteine can occur in anyone whose diet contains inadequate amounts of these vitamins. A combination of a diet high in animal protein (a source of methionine) and high in sugar and refined starch, which is consequently low in B vitamins, leads to elevated homocysteine levels and the development of atherosclerosis. Your doctor can measure your homocysteine levels with a routine blood test.

OBESITY

Have you ever tried to lose weight following any of the low-fat weight loss programs promoted in the media or even those recommended by your doctor? If so, you may have been able to lose a few pounds initially, but if you are like most people, over time the weight came right back. The end result was little or no weight loss. In fact, most people tend to not only regain the weight but add on a few extra pounds for good measure. While you were dieting, you struggled with feelings of deprivation, hunger, cravings, low energy, depression, and mood swings—all common to low-fat dieting, yet in the end it was all for naught. Why weren't you successful? It most likely had nothing to do with a lack of willpower.

The problem lies with the diet itself. Low-fat, calorie-restricted diets are doomed to fail because they are based on the erroneous belief that all calories are alike, regardless of their source. It doesn't matter if the calories come from carbohydrate, protein, or fat—a calorie is a calorie. This belief tends to single out fat because it contains more than twice as many calories as either carbohydrate or protein. One gram of carbohydrate or protein each supplies 4 calories, while a gram of fat supplies 9 calories.

If all calories are equal, it appears to make sense to cut down on fat consumption as a means to reduce total calorie intake. As a consequence, fat has been targeted as the villain and eating too much fat is often blamed for our obesity epidemic. The problem is that fat consumption has declined over the past 30 years from about 40 percent to 32 percent, but at the same time overweight and obesity have skyrocketed. If we eat less fat, why are we fatter? Something must be wrong with the theory.

Studies as far back as the 1950s have shown that people eating high-carbohydrate diets gain more weight and have more difficulty losing weight than those eating high-fat or high-protein diets with an equal number of calories, disproving the theory that the source of the calories is not important.[8]

Most overweight people don't overconsume fatty foods; in fact, just the opposite. They are the ones who are most likely to choose low-fat foods, trim the fat off of meat, and limit the amount of foods they eat. Slim people, on the other hand, generally eat whatever they please, gorging on fatty foods, and eating to their hearts' content. Those people who have a history of weight problems are more likely than normal-weight individuals to eat low-fat foods. They eat fewer calories but have greater difficulty losing and maintaining their weight.

Most of the fat in our bodies does not come from the fat in our diets; it comes from the carbohydrate we eat. The carbohydrate in our diet that is not used immediately for energy, is converted into fat and stored in our fat cells. Most of the protein and fat we consume is used as structural materials to build and maintain muscles, bones, and other tissues. Normally, only a small fraction of the protein and fat we eat is used to produce energy or is stored as fat. The body does not need to use protein and fat for energy because there is so much carbohydrate available, even an excess. This excess carbohydrate is what ends up as body fat.

When fatty foods are removed from the diet they are replaced with low-fat foods, which are typically rich in carbohydrate. This means that all low-fat diets are also high-carb diets. Because carbohydrate promotes weight gain, all low-fat diets are doomed to failure from the start.

Why does carbohydrate promote weight gain more than fat and protein? It's the glucose. As you recall from the previous chapter, after a meal, carbohydrate is converted into glucose and released into the bloodstream. As glucose levels rise, a signal is sent to release insulin. As glucose is absorbed into the cells and blood levels decline, another signal is sent to slow down the release of insulin. In this process, blood insulin and glucose levels both rise and fall in tandem.

Insulin not only shuttles glucose into the cells, but also triggers the conversion of glucose into fat and shuttles fat into the fat cells. *Insulin is a fat-storage hormone.* The more insulin you have coursing through your veins, the more fat is produced and deposited in your fat cells, and the more weight you gain.

Every time you eat carbohydrate, your blood sugar and insulin levels rise, shifting your body into fat storage mode. Protein and fat have little to no effect on blood glucose levels. Consequently, fat and protein do not stimulate much of an insulin response and do not promote weight gain.

This problem is greatly compounded when the diet includes a lot of sugars and refined starch. Such a diet promotes insulin resistance. When the cells become insulin resistant, blood sugar and insulin levels are always elevated above normal—even when nothing is being eaten. Your fasting blood sugar is a measure of how much glucose you normally have in your bloodstream when you have not eaten anything. Of course, when you do eat something, your blood sugar will rise even higher. When you have elevated blood sugar, it means you also have elevated insulin, and as long as your insulin levels are elevated, the glucose in your blood is being converted into fat and stored in the fat cells. When you are insulin resistant, this is happening continually whether you are eating or not.

When you eat too much sugar and starch, your body is programmed to store fat. Not only do increased insulin levels tell the body to store sugar as fat, they also tell it not to release any stored fat. This makes it impossible for you to use your own stored body fat for energy. So, the excess carbohydrate in your diet not only makes you fat, it makes sure you stay fat. Most low-calorie weight loss diets allow and even promote the use of refined carbohydrates, which release so much insulin that they make losing weight an arduous task, dependent on excessive calorie restriction.

Being overweight or obese isn't just about your weight and physical appearance, it profoundly affects your health. The incidence of heart disease is significantly increased in people who are overweight or obese. Obesity is defined as 20 percent or more overweight. Nearly 70 percent of the diagnosed cases of heart disease are related to obesity. The risk of death rises with increasing weight. Even moderate weight excess (10 to 20 pounds for a person of average height) increases the risk of death, particularly among adults between the ages of 30 and 64.

Body weight has a direct influence on several risk factors for heart disease. High blood pressure is twice as common in adults who are obese than in those who maintain a healthy weight. Obesity is associated with elevated blood fat levels and decreased HDL (good) cholesterol. A weight gain of only 11 to 18 pounds doubles a person's risk of developing type 2 diabetes. Insulin resistance and hyperinsulinemia (high insulin levels), which are conditions associated with diabetes, increase with weight. Over 80 percent of the people with type 2 diabetes are overweight or obese.

Not only is obesity associated with these other risk factors, but it is a risk factor in itself. Long-term studies indicate that obesity is an independent risk factor for heart disease. This relation appears to exist for both men and women with minimal increases in weight.

Obesity is a major health problem, and the primary cause is the overconsumption of sugars and refined starch, not fat.

NEURODEGENERATION: THE NEW DIABETES
Sugar Doesn't Make Memories Sweeter

One of the major benefits of cutting down on sugar consumption is better memory. Excess sugar consumption can keep you from remembering what day it is, where you live, or the name of your spouse. Compelling evidence suggests that the overconsumption of sugary foods and drinks can lead to Alzheimer's. Read that again: it's possible that sugar will cause Alzheimer's disease.

84

Studies show that excess consumption of sweet foods, particularly sugar-sweetened beverages, plays an important role in the epidemic of obesity and diabetes.[9] Diabetes—or rather, insulin resistance—is strongly associated with an increased risk of Alzheimer's disease, and evidence suggests it may also be a contributing factor in Parkinson's and other neurodegenerative diseases. Evidence is now emerging that shows a relationship between high sugar consumption and mental deterioration, learning difficulties, and memory loss.[10]

Researchers at the University of Alabama in Birmingham have shown that mice fed diets high in sugar develop the same amyloid plaque deposits in the brain and memory defects that characterize Alzheimer's disease. Over a 25-week period, one group of mice received a diet consisting of mouse chow and regular water. The other group ate the same chow, but drank a sugar water solution. The sugar-fed mice gained about 17 percent more weight over the course of the study and were more likely to develop insulin resistance—the hallmark feature of diabetes. These mice also performed worse on tests designed to measure learning and memory retention. The brains of the sugar-fed mice also showed the presence of Alzheimer's-like plaque deposits.[11]

The amount of sugar water consumed by the mice was equivalent to a human drinking five 12-ounce cans of regular soda a day. Five cans of soda contain about 180 grams of sugar. While most people don't drink five cans of soda every day, they do get sugar from other sources that can easily surpass 180 grams. On average, every man, woman, and child consumes about this much sugar every single day. Of course, an infant or a child will consume less, and some people eat almost no sugar at all, so those adults who do eat sugar are consuming well over 180 grams daily. It is interesting that the memory defects and plaque deposits in the sugar-fed mice occurred after only 25 weeks. What happens in our brains after years of eating a high-sugar diet?

Insulin Resistance and the Brain

Diabetes has long been known to adversely affect nerve tissue throughout the body, including the brain. Studies show that diabetics have substantially smaller brain volumes in comparison to nondiabetic subjects. The decrease in size is due to the death of brain cells. The brains of people with diabetes age prematurely. Sudha Seshadri, MD, a neurologist at Boston University, says that the brains of diabetics are about "10 years older" than the brains of same-age people without diabetes. Diabetics have almost twice the risk of developing Alzheimer's disease as the general population.[12] The younger a person is when he or she develops insulin resistance, the greater the risk. Even pre-diabetics are in danger of developing Alzheimer's. The common denominator between pre-diabetes, diabetes, and Alzheimer's disease is insulin resistance.

Insulin does a lot more than regulate blood sugar. Insulin plays a role in normal cognitive function. Dysregulation of insulin increases risk for cognitive impairment, Alzheimer's and other neurodegenerative diseases. Recent studies confirm that diabetes leads to a significant cognitive decline and increases the risks of dementia and Alzheimer's disease by up to 150 percent.[13]

Not only does insulin resistance increase the risk of Alzheimer's, it appears to be essential for the development of the disease. In fact, Alzheimer's is now recognized as a form of diabetes—brain diabetes. It is referred to as type 3 diabetes. Type 2 and type 3 diabetes often occur together, but not always. All Alzheimer's patients have elevated whole-body insulin resistance, but in some cases it is not elevated enough to be classified as type 2 diabetes. All Alzheimer's patients, however, have severely altered brain glucose metabolism—brain insulin resistance.

Other neurological disorders, such as vascular dementia, Parkinson's disease, Huntington's disease, and ALS, also exhibit features suggesting insulin resistance as either an important underlying factor or as a contributor to the initiation and progression of these diseases.[14-16] All of the major neurodegenerative diseases display a marked decline in energy metabolism, leading to cell death and loss of brain volume. Any disturbance in normal insulin function can dramatically affect energy metabolism and consequently brain function. In that sense, they might all be viewed as various manifestations of type 3 diabetes.

Having diabetes is known to increase the risk of developing Parkinson's. In one of the largest studies of its kind to date, researchers followed a group of more than 50,000 men and women over a period of 18 years. The researchers found that those people who had type 2 diabetes at the start of the study were 83 percent more likely to be diagnosed with Parkinson's disease later on in life than nondiabetics.[17] There appears to be a strong connection between Parkinson's and insulin resistance.[18] Abnormal glucose tolerance has been reported in up to 80 percent of Parkinson's disease patients. Dysfunction of insulin metabolism in the brain is known to precede the death of the dopamine-producing neurons in the development of Parkinson's disease.[19] Insulin resistance also exacerbates the severity of the symptoms and reduces the therapeutic efficacy of drug therapy.[20]

Amyotrophic lateral sclerosis, or ALS, is a brain disorder that affects the motor neurons that control the muscles of the body. ALS causes the muscle to atrophy, leading to paralysis and eventually death. Since the 1950s insulin resistance has been reported in a significant percentage of patients with ALS.[21]

Even Huntington's disease, a degenerative brain disorder that is considered primarily an inherited condition, also appears to be influenced by insulin resistance. Studies show that those with Huntington's disease are more likely to have diabetes than those without the disease.[22-23]

The changes that take place in the body that lead to diabetes and eventually to neurodegeneration occur long before these diseases become apparent. Glucose metabolism becomes abnormal one to two decades before type 2 diabetes is diagnosed. Neurodegenerative disease may surface another couple of decades after that.

Diabetes is on the rise. According to the Mayo Clinic, diabetes has doubled in the United States over the past 15 years. Worldwide diabetes has increased from 30 million to 230 million cases over the past 20 years. This is a huge increase. Scientists have expressed concern that today's mushrooming diabetes epidemic may become tomorrow's Alzheimer's epidemic or Parkinson's epidemic. The epidemic may have already begun—as witnessed by the increasing rates of Alzheimer's, Parkinson's, and other neurodegenerative diseases. For example, as much as 80 percent of tissues involved may be damaged before a person can be diagnosed with Alzheimer's or Parkinson's disease.

If you are having memory or cognitive problems or feel you are losing your mind to neurodegeneration, you likely have sugar to thank for it.

Eye Health

The eyes are extensions of the brain. Anything that affects the brain also affects the eyes. High blood sugar profoundly affects eye health. People with diabetes often experience blurred vision, since high blood sugar initiates degenerative changes in the blood vessels in the retina—the photosensitive cells at the back of the eye that relay visual messages to the brain. Blurred vision may, in fact, be the first sign of diabetes. One of the major complications of insulin resistance is diabetic retinopathy, which is the slow degeneration of the retina. There is no question that insulin resistance threatens vision; patients with diabetes develop cataracts at an earlier age and are nearly twice as likely to develop glaucoma as compared to nondiabetics.

The longer a person has diabetes, the more likely he or she is to develop retinopathy. Almost everyone with type 1 diabetes and most of those with type 2 diabetes will eventually develop retinopathy. Nearly half of those diagnosed with diabetes already have some stage of retinopathy. In most Western countries diabetic retinopathy is the leading cause of blindness in individuals ages 20 to 65.

If you have problems with cataracts, glaucoma, macular degeneration, or any other age-related eye disorder, you are most likely insulin resistant, at least to some degree. As one example, the higher a person's blood sugar

87

is, the greater the risk of cataract. Researchers at Yale University studied the effects of three diets—high-carb, high-protein, and high-fat—on the incidence of cataracts in diabetic rats. As expected, blood sugar levels were highest on the high-carb diet and lowest on the high-fat diet. Development of cataracts was highest in the rats fed a high-carb diet; a lesser incidence was observed in the high-protein fed animals, while no cataracts developed in rats fed a high-fat diet.[24] Although all the rats in this study were diabetic, their diets—not the disease—determined the level of cataracts they developed. The higher the blood sugar levels, the greater the incidence of cataracts. When blood sugar was controlled by a high-fat, low-carb diet, no cataracts developed. This effect is similar in humans, as better blood sugar control has shown similar results.[25]

Whether you are diabetic or not, eating a high-carb diet will elevate blood sugar and keep it elevated for extended periods of time, increasing your risk of damage to the brain and eyes. Scientists working for the U.S. Agricultural Research Service tracked 471 middle-aged women over a 14-year period. The researchers found that the women with an average daily carbohydrate intake, between 200 and 268 grams, typical for most women of normal weight, were 2.5 times more likely to get cataracts than those who consumed between 101 and 185 grams per day. Although the consumption of 101 to 185 grams per day is lower than average, it is not considered low-carb. Low-carb diets generally include no more than 100 grams of carbohydrate a day, and very low-carb diets restrict it to fewer than 30 grams. We can conclude from this research that even a modest reduction in carbohydrate intake, and the corresponding drop in blood sugar levels, can significantly reduce risk of cataracts.[26]

Fasting blood sugar measures the glucose levels at the time of testing. Another way of measuring blood sugar is the A1C test, which gives an average over the previous three months. Researchers at the University of Oxford found that type 2 diabetics who lower their A1C level by just 1 percent can reduce their risk of cataracts by 19 percent.[27] It appears that even a small decrease in average blood sugar can make a big impact on eye health.

The Diabetes Control and Complications Trial (DCCT) showed that better control of blood sugar levels also substantially slows the onset and progression of retinopathy.[28] Diabetics who kept their blood sugar levels as close to normal as possible also had much less kidney and nerve disease. Better control also reduces the need for sight-saving laser surgery.

Blood sugar levels increase the risk and progression of macular degeneration. According to the University of Illinois Eye and Ear Infirmary, one serving per day of processed baked goods (e.g., a slice of bread, a bagel, pie, cake, or cookie) increases risk of macular degeneration progression by

2.42 times. On the flipside, simply reducing your intake of high-carb foods by one serving per day can reduce your risk by 2.42 times.

Elevated blood sugar levels, even those considered within typical or average range, accelerates brain aging and degeneration.[29] Any chronic elevation of blood sugar is harmful to the eyes, so even those with so-called normal fasting glucose levels may be at increased risk. If your fasting glucose levels are above 90 mg/dl, you are at risk, and the higher the level, the greater that risk.

The bitter truth is that you may be at risk of developing an age-related eye disease, even if you have no known visual difficulties; we are all at risk. As with the brain, degenerative diseases of the eyes don't appear overnight; rather, they take years, even decades to develop. Glucose metabolism becomes abnormal one to two decades before type 2 diabetes is diagnosed.[30] In the meantime, the damage done can be extensive, long before any symptoms become noticeable. Since no pain or sudden changes in vision are noticed, the gradual loss of sight is not easily recognized until substantial damage has occurred. Even though you may not notice any serious problem with your vision now, it is possible that your eyes have already experienced some degree of abnormal degeneration. If you wait until symptoms become noticeable, it may be too late to fully correct the problem.

Unlike the brain, which is inaccessible and not easily observed, the eyes can be carefully examined without too much difficulty. Your eye doctor can tell if you are developing a problem, oftentimes before it is too late. For this reason, it is a good idea to have your eyes examined periodically. Also, you should have your fasting blood glucose levels checked every few years. If your blood sugar is high, take steps now to correct the problem and you will greatly reduce your risk of experiencing vision loss later on.

DIGESTIVE HEALTH

The foods you eat not only affect your health but also the health of the microorganisms that live in your digestive tract—some 100 trillion of them. The health of these tiny organisms may not seem to be of much significance, but their health has a direct impact on your health. These organisms play an essential role in keeping us healthy and disease-free. They help maintain pH balance of the digestive tract; synthesize important vitamins, such as vitamins B_{12} and K; support immune function; aid in the breakdown and digestion of food; neutralize toxins; regulate glucose absorption and metabolism; and protect against inflammatory diseases and the colonization of pathogenic organisms.

This community of microorganisms, known as the gut *microbiome*, is highly diverse, consisting of some 10,000 to 30,000 different species of bacteria, viruses, and fungi. Individual species of this inner ecology are referred to as the *microbiota*.

Disruption of this carefully balanced population of microbes has been implicated as a contributing factor in many health problems, including obesity, insulin resistance and diabetes, reduced immune function, digestive disorders (chronic constipation, inflammatory bowel diseases, celiac disease), neurological disorders (Alzheimer's, Parkinson's, autism, ADHD, depression), food allergies and sensitivities, eczema, recurrent yeast problems, and some forms of cancer. The health of our digestive system is so important that it has been said that up to 90 percent of all known human illness can be traced back to an unhealthy gut.

The term "gut" refers to the gastrointestinal system, which extends from the mouth to the rectum. When food is swallowed, its first stop is in the stomach, where it is mixed with digestive enzymes and stomach acids. From there it goes into the upper end of the small intestine, which consists of a 1-inch-diameter (2.5 cm) tube that is about 23 feet long. The lower end of the small intestine is attached to the large intestine (also called the colon), which is only about 5 feet long. Although much shorter than the small intestine, the colon is referred to as the large intestine because it is fatter, about 3 inches (7.5 cm) in diameter. It is in the large intestine that the vast majority of our microbiota reside.

Our diet has a profound effect on the types of organisms that live in our digestive tract, and therefore, on our digestive function and overall health. The foods we eat are the foods our microbiota eats. Like us, these microorganisms have preferences: some prefer sugar and simple carbohydrates while others prefer more complex carbohydrates, indigestible dietary fiber, or other food components. The population of the sugar lovers blooms when we eat a lot of sugary foods or highly refined processed grains. In contrast, the fiber lovers are happiest when the diet is rich in vegetables, fruits, whole grains, nuts, and seeds. Sugar and refined starch encourage the growth of undesirable microbiota that provide little benefit and have the potential to cause trouble. When the diet is loaded with sugar and refined carbohydrate, these undesirable microbes thrive, crowding out more useful, health-promoting organisms that prefer more complex carbohydrates. A diet heavy in sugar is consequently low in fiber. This results in a serious imbalance in the gut microbiome.

Fiber is often viewed as an indigestible, and otherwise nearly useless, food component, yet it is extremely important for good digestive function and overall health. It softens the stool, shortens transit time through the intestinal tract, slows down the absorption of glucose, helps balance the pH, and absorbs and removes certain toxins, preventing them from entering the bloodstream. Most important, however, is that it provides food for our resident gut microbiota. While the human body does not possess the enzymes needed to breakdown or digest fiber, our gut bacteria do. Fiber-loving bacteria feed on it, and in the process the fiber is transformed into short chain fatty acids (SCFAs). These SCFAs serve as food for the layer of cells lining the digestive tract (the epithelium). Most of the fiber-loving bacteria live in the colon. SCFAs are the primary energy source for the epithelial cells in the colon and supply 60 to 70 percent of their energy needs. A lack of dietary fiber can seriously affect the populations of the SCFA-producing bacteria, and consequently, the health of the colon itself.

SCFAs are important to the health of your intestines and the integrity of the intestinal wall. Without them, the epithelial cells lining the digestive tract would begin to degenerate; they would literally starve to death. This would cause chronic inflammation and tissue breakdown, which could lead to leaky gut syndrome, lesions or ulcers, diverticulitis, ulcerative colitis, Crohn's disease, irritable bowel syndrome, and other digestive disorders. Nutrient absorption could also be dramatically affected, leading to malnutrition. Evidence suggests that many people suffering from inflammatory bowel diseases are really suffering from a malnourished digestive tract.

Our modern diet is woefully deficient in dietary fiber. Sugar contains no fiber. Refined grains are almost completely devoid of it. Processed flours and sugar make up about 50 percent of the calories in the average diet. The small amount of fiber in the diet may be enough to keep the intestinal cells from total starvation, but not healthy. A diet lacking an adequate amount of high-fiber foods can lead to various forms of digestive distress as well as malnutrition.

SCFAs do much more than just provide food for intestinal epithelial cells. Recent research reveals that they play a key role in the prevention and treatment of metabolic syndrome, insulin resistance and diabetes, bowel disorders, osteoporosis, kidney disease, hypertension, and colon cancer.[31-34] SCFAs lower the colonic pH (i.e., raises the acidity level in the colon), which provides a suitable environment for helpful microbiota, protects the lining from forming colonic polyps, and increases absorption of dietary minerals. They stimulate the production of T-helper cells, leukocytes, and antibodies that play crucial roles in immune protection. They have anti-inflammatory effects and can help ease inflammation in the digestive tract caused by microbiota dysbiosis, ulcers, injuries, and such. In clinical studies SCFAs have been used therapeutically for the successful treatment of ulcerative colitis, Crohn's disease, and antibiotic-associated diarrhea.[35-37]

ORAL HEALTH
Bacteria Feed on Sugar

The most obvious and widely recognized consequence of consuming sugar is dental decay. Even the sugar industry admits that eating too much sugary food contributes to dental decay. They can't deny it; the scientific evidence is too overwhelming. However, that's as much as they will admit, and insist that good dental hygiene—brushing and flossing daily—will prevent any problems.

We have billions of bacteria, viruses, and fungi living in our mouths. There are more than 600 species of bacteria alone that make our mouths their home. Many of these bacteria produce acids and toxins as by-products, which damage the teeth and irritate the gums, causing inflammation and bleeding. An overgrowth of these bacteria leads to tooth decay and periodontal disease (gum disease), and eventually tooth loss. Discolored teeth, plaque (bacteria colonies), calculus (calcified plaque), cavities, bleeding gums, sensitive teeth, and chronic bad breath are all signs of an overgrowth. The bacteria that cause the greatest harm feed on sugar. The more sugar we eat, the more these bacteria multiply and grow, outnumbering other, less troublesome species. It is the imbalance in the oral microbiome that is the primary cause of poor oral health.

While we all recognize that eating sugary foods can rot our teeth, little more is ever said about it. The damage sugar does to our teeth is taken for granted and brushed off as if it were inconsequential. The message we get is that brushing with fluoride toothpaste and regular professional dental care will take care of the problem, no need to worry, so eat what you want. A rotten tooth is drilled, filled, and capped—problem fixed. No steps are taken to address or correct the root cause of the problem—the oral microbiome. Cosmetic dentistry is just a temporary fix; it looks good but is not a solution. The cause of the problem has not been addressed and still exists, and over time will likely affect other teeth. If a tooth is too far destroyed by decay or gum disease, it is pulled. Consequently, despite daily brushing, millions of people wear dentures or have dental implants to replace these missing teeth.

According to the US Centers for Disease Control and Prevention (CDC), nine out of every 10 people have tooth decay. Tooth loss has become an epidemic: 1 in 20 middle-aged adults and 1 in 3 older adults over the age of 65 have lost *all* of their natural teeth to tooth decay or gum disease. This is not 2 or 3 teeth we're talking about, but all 32 adult teeth! These adult teeth, in contrast to baby or temporary teeth, are referred to as "permanent" teeth because they are supposed to last a lifetime, not just a few decades.

Dental disease starts early. Five percent of babies have some tooth decay by 9 months of age, 15 percent by 12 months, and 17 percent by 4 years of age. Parents often feed their children sugar-sweetened juices and baby foods.

When they get older, they continue with sugary junk foods. Consequently, moderate periodontal disease is found in 40 percent of children over 12 year of age. The problem usually gets worse as they get older.

The Most Prevalent Disease

Because of the wide distribution and availability of sugar and sweetened foods, oral disease is found worldwide and is the most prevalent microbial disease of mankind. According to a study in the British medical journal the *Lancet*, periodontal disease affects up to 90 percent of the population worldwide.[38] It wasn't always like this; while tooth decay and gum disease have afflicted humans throughout history, these conditions were much less frequent in ages past. The remains of ancient humans show far less oral disease than we have today..

Hunter-gatherer societies that ate high-fat diets had the least amount of dental disease. As people transitioned to agriculture, dental disease increased. Weston A. Price, DDS, observed the same thing during his ten-year study of non-modernized native populations. Those people who ate primarily meat and fat, such as the Inuit and the Native Americans, had very little tooth decay. Those populations that consumed more grains, fruits, and starchy vegetables had significantly more decay. But even then, without sugar or refined flour, their dental health was far superior to those consuming modern foods.

Because of the difference in oral infections in ancient and modern humans, scientists wanted to know if the oral bacteria today are any different from those of our distant ancestors. Oral bacteria do not survive on the teeth of ancient human remains. However, where hardened calculus is present, the oral bacteria is encased and preserved like a fossil in limestone. From these teeth it is learned that ancient humans harbored a much more diverse variety of oral microorganisms than we do today. We tend to have larger populations of the more virulent species of bacteria, such as *Streptococcus mutans*—the major cause of tooth decay. Our ancestors had *Streptococcus mutans* as well, but in such small numbers that they generally were not a problem.

We don't have to go back to ancient times to find healthy, relatively disease-free teeth. There are a few hunter-gatherer populations still living in Africa and elsewhere who eat their traditional, sugar-free diets. They have remarkably good oral health, free of gum disease and dental decay. None of them ever brush or floss their teeth. They totally ignore any attempt at oral hygiene, yet still have far better oral health than we do. However, once they start to add sugar or white flour into their diets, oral health sharply declines.

The bacteria that inhabit our mouths form a clear, sticky film on our teeth and gums, known as *dental plaque*. This layer of bacteria is constantly forming on the teeth and is actually beneficial, as it prevents acids in foods

93

from dissolving the enamel in our teeth and helps keep our teeth strong and resistant to decay. However, plaque can become harmful if it is created by the wrong type of bacteria—the bacteria that thrive on sugar.

Sugar feeds many forms of oral bacteria, such as *Streptococcus mutans*, that produce acid as a waste product. Starch also feeds these bacteria, as it is easily broken down into sugar by enzymes in saliva. If the diet contains a large amount of sugar or starch, the plaque that coats the teeth is heavily populated with these acid-forming bacteria. The acid they produce on the tooth surface dissolves the enamel, making the teeth soft and easily accessible to invasion by bacteria and other microorganisms, leading to tooth decay and possibly the loss of the tooth. This is why we are instructed to brush our teeth regularly, to scrape off the potentially harmful plaque.

Because bacteria are always present in the mouth, new plaque will immediately start to coat the teeth, so brushing must be done often. This plaque is only harmful if the diet contains excessive amounts of sugar or starch, which requires regular brushing and dental care. Ancient humans never brushed their teeth, flossed, or used antiseptic mouthwash. They didn't need to because they didn't eat sugary foods that would stimulate the growth of acid-forming bacteria. The bacteria in their mouths were less virulent, and the plaque that formed on their teeth was protective, not harmful.

The plaque that coats the teeth is a natural protective process seen in all animals. It is only when the diet is out of balance with nature that trouble arises. We are not born with teeth that are genetically designed to rot away without regular brushing and modern dental care. Animals in the wild don't need to brush their teeth or go to the dentist for regular cleanings or fillings. Our pets, however, are not so lucky. Dogs and cats, which by nature are carnivores, often develop dental problems as a result of eating high-carb, grain-based pet foods. Dental disease is a modern epidemic brought on by the overconsumption of sugar and starch.

Today we have state-of-the-art dental techniques and highly trained dentists, the best-formulated toothpastes and mouthwashes, fluoridated water, dental floss, and numerous other products and procedures to keep our teeth clean and strong, yet we have the poorest dental health of any generation in history. We also consume more sugar than any generation in history.

Oral infections are not trivial matters that can be corrected simply by more brushing or cosmetic dentistry. A bright white smile does not equate to a disease-free mouth. Appearances can be deceiving. If you have or have had any cavities or gum disease as evidenced by the presence of fillings, crowns, root canals, implants, and dentures, you most likely have an active infection right now, or at least an overgrowth of potentially harmful bacteria living in your mouth, regardless of how pearly white your teeth may be. Bleaching, straightening, and filling do not get rid of the disease-causing bacteria.

Many people may ask what's so bad about having a few cavities. All we need to do is take better care of our mouths by brushing more often; use fluoride toothpaste, floss, and mouthwash; and visit the dentist. That should solve the problem. That's what most people believe, and if you have a dental problem it is because you weren't diligent enough with your oral hygiene routine or didn't visit the dentist often enough. It is rarely blamed on the diet.

A Source of Systemic Disease

Most people have the mistaken belief that the mouth is an isolated compartment of the body and that what goes on there has no effect on the rest of the body. This belief is absolutely wrong. Your mouth is part of your digestive tract and a gateway into the body. An infection there has ample opportunity to spread throughout the body. Any oral infection, or even an overpopulation of potentially virulent microbes in the mouth, can affect your overall health. Bacteria in the mouth can seep into the bloodstream and travel throughout the body, affecting any organ or tissue in the body. This migration of microorganisms is intensified whenever an active infection is present. For this reason, oral infections can be the cause of any number of health problems, many of which are generally considered unrelated to oral health.

For example, oral infections have been linked to a number of common health problems including high blood pressure, heart disease, dementia, asthma, arthritis, colitis, osteoporosis, diabetes, and numerous infectious illnesses.[39-44]

Our oral health can even affect the health of our unborn children. Periodontal or gum disease can adversely affect pregnancy outcome, increasing the risk of delivering preterm and low birth weight babies.[45] Research shows that pregnant women with periodontal disease are seven and a half times more likely to have a premature or underweight delivery, and the more severe the disease, the greater effect it has on the baby. An infant's birth weight is the most potent single indicator of the infant's health status. A low birth weight baby has a statistically greater chance of developing diseases and of dying early in life.

The risk of oral bacteria spreading to other parts of the body is very real and potentially serious. If you have had any heart problems, when you visit the dentist, he or she will prescribe antibiotics for you before working on your mouth, because even routine dental work will likely cause small lacerations in the gums that will allow large amounts of bacteria into your bloodstream that can go to the heart and possibly cause heart failure. There is a very strong relationship between cardiovascular disease and oral health. Having poor oral health greatly increases your risk of having a heart attack or stroke.

If microorganisms that normally inhabit the mouth find their way into the bloodstream, they can infect artery walls, causing localized low-grade infections and chronic inflammation. In this manner, bacteria and viruses can cause atherosclerosis, which can lead to heart attacks and strokes. The connection between infections and atherosclerosis is strengthened by the fact that fragments of bacteria are often found inside arterial plaque. Brent Muhlestein, a cardiologist at the LDS Hospital in Salt Lake City and the University of Utah, has found that 79 percent of plaque specimens taken from the coronary arteries of 90 heart disease patients showed the presence of bacteria. In addition, researchers have also found live oral bacteria, the smoking gun as you might say, in arterial plaque, thus demonstrating its involvement in the plaque-forming process.[46] This supplies the proof that live bacteria from the oral cavity have become inhabitants of the artery wall.

The bacteria and viruses that cause periodontal disease are known to cause atherosclerosis in animals and have also been found in human arterial plaque.[47] Studies have shown that heart disease patients have more tooth decay and higher rates of gum disease than the general population.[48] For example, Robert J. Genco, DDS, PhD, of the University of Buffalo, studied 1,372 people over a 10-year period and found that heart disease was three times more prevalent for those with gum disease.[49] In the National Health and Nutritional Examination Study, people with inflammation of the gums had a 25 percent increased risk of heart disease.[50] The risk was high even for those who had gum disease in the past as well as currently, indicating that gum disease may not have been completely resolved. They also found that the more severe the periodontal disease, the greater the risk of developing heart disease.

Studies indicate that people with periodontal disease have a 200 percent increased risk of dying from cardiovascular disease.[51] This is astronomical. By comparison, smokers only have a 60 percent increased risk. The presence of periodontal disease is a far more accurate indicator of heart disease risk than smoking. Tooth decay and gum disease have now become recognized as being more strongly associated with coronary heart disease than any of the standard recognized risk factors, namely, blood cholesterol levels, being overweight, diabetes, sedentary lifestyle, and smoking.[52]

Diabetes is another condition that is related to poor dental health. Periodontal infections can promote insulin resistance. Pro-inflammatory chemicals released in response to infection or injury desensitize cells to insulin. Untreated periodontal disease causes chronic inflammation, which in turn can increase systemic insulin resistance, promoting diabetes or exacerbating the condition if it already exists.[53-54] Treating periodontal disease and improving oral health has shown to improve systemic insulin resistance.[55]

Diabetes is commonly diagnosed by chronic elevated blood sugar levels. The glucose levels in saliva mirror those of the blood. Generally, oral bacteria will feed on sugar when we eat, and for a limited time afterwards. In the case of a diabetic, blood glucose is always elevated above normal; this causes saliva glucose to be continually elevated, allowing for the bacteria in the mouth to be feeding and multiplying nonstop even when food is not being consumed. For this reason, diabetics are very prone to tooth decay and gum disease. This in turn can cause diabetes to worsen because the infection allows more bacteria to enter the bloodstream, causing systemic inflammation, which promotes insulin resistance. Diabetes promotes oral infections and oral infections promote diabetes—it's a vicious cycle causing the diabetes to get worse. Dentists can often diagnose diabetes just from examining the condition of a patient's mouth.

The level of glucose in saliva is consistent with the level in the blood, and for this reason, measuring glucose levels in saliva has been suggested as an alternative method of testing for blood glucose levels in determining insulin resistance and diagnosing diabetes.[56]

The condition of your teeth and gums may affect your mind as well. Research is linking Alzheimer's and Parkinson's disease to oral health. Alzheimer's and dementia patients have, in general, poor oral health.[57-58] Patients suffering from dementia have twice the number of dental cavities as age-matched people with normal mental function. Parkinson's patients also suffer from an increased incidence of tooth decay, periodontal disease, and tooth loss.[59] In some cases, the onset of Parkinson's disease has been linked directly to bacteria overgrowth and periodontal disease.[60]

Periodontal disease is the most common cause of tooth loss in adults. Generally, missing teeth indicate a history of poor oral health and bacteria overgrowth. The fewer teeth a person has, the greater the likelihood of developing neurodegenerative disease.

A team of researchers from the University of Kentucky College of Medicine and College of Dentistry investigated the relationships between tooth loss, dementia, and Alzheimer's in what is known as the Nun Study. The study included 144 Catholic nuns ranging in age from 75 to 98. The researchers analyzed dental records and the results of annual cognitive examinations over a period of ten years. Autopsy findings were also used for 118 of the participants who died during the study period. The researchers found that those with the fewest teeth at the beginning of the study were the most likely to develop dementia. This study demonstrated that the more teeth removed due to poor dental health, the greater the risk of dementia.[61]

To rule out possible genetic factors, researchers investigated the relationship between tooth loss and dementia among identical twins. Participants included 106 pairs of identical twins age 65 or older, with one twin from each pair suffering from dementia. Investigators discovered that a history of tooth loss, particularly before age 35, was a significant risk factor for Alzheimer's disease.[62] This study not only showed that oral health is a risk factor for dementia, but that the processes associated with dental health that lead to dementia start earlier in life. A person's dental health in the prime of life can affect his or her mental health in later years.

The health of your mouth is not a trivial matter; it can affect the health of your entire body. Poor oral health can be a direct cause, or at least a contributing factor, in the development of many chronic conditions. There is a greater connection between heart disease and oral health (and sugar consumption) than there is to dietary fat intake. Oral health is directly related to diet, and it is primarily sugar and refined starch that promote the over-growth of bacteria that infect the teeth and gums. In this manner, sugar can be an indirect but highly significant cause of many of our chronic illnesses.

IMMUNE FUNCTION AND CANCER

We live in an environment surrounded by potentially harmful bacteria, parasites, and other microorganisms. They are in the food we eat, the water we drink, and the air we breathe. In addition, we are assaulted continually by environmental and industrial toxins; even our own bodies produce toxic products such as AGEs and free radicals. On top of that, damaged, defective, and diseased cells are scattered throughout our bodies. With all this going on, it's amazing we can survive. Fortunately, our bodies have a way of cleaning up this mess and protecting us from harm. That job is handled by our immune system.

We have many immune cells, but it is the army of white blood cells patrolling our bodies that spearhead our defense. These cells combat potentially harmful substances in a variety of ways. One of the most important is a process called *phagocytosis*. This is a process in which white blood cells consume and digest any foreign or defective cells.

The ability of white blood cells to do this, however, is strongly influenced by sugar consumption. Sugar depresses the white blood cells' ability to phagocytize these harmful substances. Studies have shown that after a single dose of sugar, phagocytosis drops by nearly 50 percent and remains depressed for up to five hours.[63] If you eat a sugary meal, your immune system will be severely depressed and will likely remain that way until your next meal. So, if you eat pancakes or sugary breakfast cereal in the morning, drink a sugary soda with your lunch, and end your dinner with a bowl of ice cream, your immune system will be severely depressed all day long.

You will be less able to remove invading microorganisms, toxins, AGEs, and renegade cells (cancer).

Because sugar depresses immune function, it increases the risks of infection, reduces the body's ability to neutralize and dispose of environmental toxins, and increases the risk of cancer. Consequently, you become more susceptible to infectious disease, have a more difficult time overcoming infections, are more vulnerable or sensitive to toxins and chemicals, and are more likely to develop cancer.

One out of every three people alive today in the United States will eventually get some form of cancer during his or her lifetime. Cancer is second only to heart disease as the leading cause of death in the world. This isn't so shocking when you realize that every single one of us has cancerous cells in our bodies. These renegade cells are just a part of our biology and its interaction with the environment. The reason we don't all develop cancer and die is because the immune system seeks out and destroys these renegade cells before they can get too far out of hand. As long as the immune system is functioning as it should, we need not worry about cancer. Arthur I. Holleb, MD, senior vice president of Medical Affairs for the American Cancer Society, stated, "Only when the immune system is incapable of destroying these malignant cells will cancer develop."[64] In other words, cancer can only develop in those individuals whose immune systems are so stressed or weakened that they are incapable of mounting an effective defense. Dr. Holleb didn't specify only lung cancer or breast cancer or leukemia as being affected by the immune system's efficiency. He referred to all cancers, which means that even if we are exposed to carcinogenic substances, if the immune system is working as it should, cancer will not develop. A healthy immune system, therefore, is a key element in the prevention of all forms of cancer.

One of the major causes of chronic stress on the immune system is its constant battle with the bacteria seeping into our bloodstream from our mouths. This problem is compounded when an oral infection is present. Sugar both promotes chronic oral infections and depresses the immune system, making it easier for cancer to take a foothold. Consequently, periodontal disease and tooth loss greatly increase the risk of many forms of cancer,[65-69] most notably, esophageal, upper gastrointestinal, gastric, colorectal, lung, bladder, prostate, and pancreatic cancers, as well as melanoma, non-Hodgkin 's lymphoma, leukemia, and multiple myeloma.[70]

If your immune system is depressed from a high-sugar diet, cancer is given the green light to grow and multiply. To make matters worse, the sugar acts as a fertilizer to the cancer. Cancer cells feed on sugar. The more sugar you feed them, the heartier they grow.[71]

One of the differences between healthy cells and cancerous cells is in the production of energy. The cell organelles (cell organs) that are primarily involved in energy metabolism are the mitochondria. The mitochondria are adaptable and can use a variety of nutrients to produce energy. In cancer cells, however, the mitochondria are defective and are unable to produce energy. This requires cancer cells to rely on another means of energy production, called *glycolysis*, which does not involve the mitochondria.

The glucose in our blood is essential for glycolysis. Fatty acids, ketones, and most other energy sources are useless to cancer cells. This makes cancer heavily reliant on glucose for its energy needs. The more sugar you supply them, from a diet filled with sugary foods and refined starch, the more energy they have available, the quicker they grow, and the more resistant they become to cancer treatments. On the other hand, without sugar they would starve to death and be far more vulnerable to the immune system and to cancer treatments.

Insulin resistance and high blood glucose are considered to be independent risk factors for cancer. The association between diabetes, particularly type 2 diabetes, and cancer is well recognized. Studies show that people with diabetes are at substantially higher risk of cancer, especially of the pancreas, liver, lung, endometrium, breast, colon, rectum, and bladder.[72]

Insulin resistance means constantly elevated blood sugar so that there is more blood sugar flowing through the veins than normal. This sugar feeds cancer.

The fact that cancer feeds almost exclusively on sugar and needs lots of it has been used for many years in medical imaging. Positron emission tomography (PET) scans are a useful tool to detect cancer. The patient is given a sugary drink with radioactive ions. The cancer will immediately "eat" the sugar and get a dose of radioactive ions. The PET scan shows the areas of the body with heightened glucose metabolism, indicating the presence of cancer. Cancer acts as a glucose magnet.

Sugar feeds all forms of cancer. Smoking has long been believed to be the primary cause of lung cancer. Men who smoke are 23 times more likely to develop lung cancer and women are 13 times more likely, compared to those who have never smoked. Secondhand smoke is nearly as bad; nonsmokers who are exposed to secondhand smoke at home or work have a 20 to 30 percent greater risk of developing this type of cancer.

Lung cancer is the most common cancer worldwide, accounting for 2.1 million new cases and 1.8 million deaths per year in 2018. It is by far the leading cause of cancer death among both men and women. Each year, more people die from lung cancer than from colon, breast, and prostate cancer combined.[73]

While there is no question that smoking contributes to lung cancer and many other health problems, it may not be the primary factor involved. Diet and blood sugar appears to play a significant role. The correlation between

100

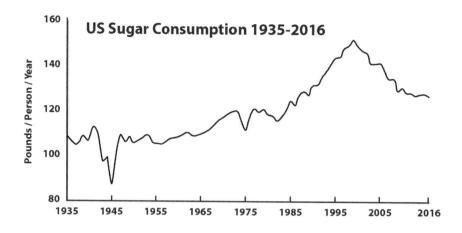

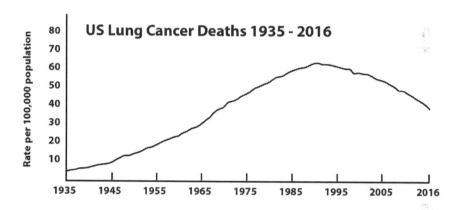

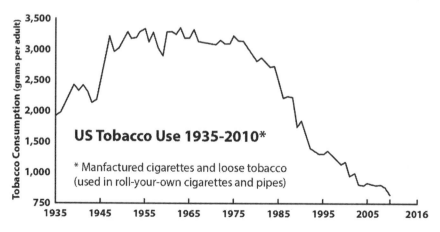

Source: US Department of Agriculture, American Cancer Society, and American Lung Association.

lung cancer deaths and sugar consumption is striking (see the graphs on the previous page). Sugar consumption has risen steadily and peaked in 1999 and then has gradually declined. Lung cancer has followed the same general pattern. In contrast, the correlation between tobacco use and lung cancer is not as obvious. In the United States, the use of tobacco products has been declining since the 1970s, tobacco use is lower now than it has been in a century, yet lung cancer deaths are as high now as they were in the 1970s. If smoking causes cancer, why did lung cancer deaths continue to rise and remain high while tobacco use has dramatically declined?

It is quite possible that smoking, by itself, may not be enough to cause cancer. Sugar may the catalyst that makes tobacco so dangerous.

Prior to the mid-1900s, lung cancer was relatively uncommon in the US. In 1930 the death rate due to lung cancer for both men and women was less than 3.5 per 100,000 population. In 2016 the rate for men was 46.7 and women 31.9 per 100,000.[74] The number of smokers has decreased while lung cancer deaths have increase over tenfold. There has to be something else going on here.

Smoking has never been a major problem in any population until sugar and refined flour have been added to the diet. Many primitive societies have used tobacco for generations without suffering any apparent harm. For example, the Inuit of northern Canada and Alaska have traditionally been very heavy smokers. Despite the fact that they lived a nomadic hunter-gatherer lifestyle, they obtained tobacco through trade. Nearly all Inuit smoked. Every evening they would go into their shelters, which were tightly sealed off from the bitter arctic cold, and smoke. The room would fill with tobacco smoke as well as smoke from the fires that keep them warm and gave them light, with only one small air vent in the middle of the roof. Everyone, including young children, were exposed to heavy doses of secondhand smoke.

The smoking habits of the Inuit were recorded by many of the arctic explorers. In the early 1900s, anthropologist Vilhjalmur Stefansson, described their habitual use of tobacco. If smoking caused lung cancer, the Inuit would definitely have had a cancer epidemic. However, one of the things Stefansson noted was the complete absence of cancer of any type.[75] A diet rich in fruits and vegetables was not what was protecting them. At that time, the Inuit diet consisted almost entirely of meat and fat. They ate no vegetables, fruits, or grains and absolutely no sugar or sweets of any kind, except what little they might obtain on rare occasions from isolated trading posts.

Dr. Otto Schaefer, who attended to the medical needs of the Inuit and Native Americans in the Canadian Arctic from the mid-1950s to the late 1960s reported that cancer was not found among these people until after they began to add sugar and refined carbohydrates into their diets. Lung cancer was completely absent among them. Dr. Schaefer observed that smoking itself did not cause cancer in the Inuit unless the diet also included sugar. "If smoking alone causes lung cancer," wrote Dr. Schaefer, "we should expect to find many cases of Eskimos and Indians, who almost all smoke quite heavily, mostly cigarettes in recent decades. No bronchogenic cancer had been found [among the natives of Northern Canada.]"[76]

The absence of lung cancer is not unique to the Inuit and Native Americans, but has been observed in many primitive cultures throughout the world that ate a sugar-free diet.

Even in our own culture, we have known or heard of people who smoked and yet lived long healthy lives, free of cancer. A good example is the cigar smoking actor and comedian George Burns. He began smoking at the age of 14 and is reported to have smoked between 10 and 15 cigars a day for over 70 years (more than 300,000 cigars in his lifetime). Burns remained in good health all his life and was still actively working as a stand-up comedian until just weeks before his death in 1996, at the ripe old age of 100. He exercised regularly, was not overweight, did not have any blood sugar problems, and ate a relatively low-sugar diet. He even wrote a bestselling diet book titled *How to Live to Be 100—Or More*. Despite his heavy smoking, his diet and lifestyle had the greater influence on his health.

Smoking is not benign by any means; it is a risk factor for a multitude of diseases. However, it appears that smoking itself is not enough to cause lung cancer until it is combined with a poor diet high in sugar. It appears to be the tobacco-sugar one-two punch that is the real culprit in causing lung cancer. Sugar is likely the catalyst for other cancers as well.

Glucose is so important to the growth of cancer that it can't survive without it. Removing sugar and other carbohydrates from the diet essentially starves cancer to death. Dietary therapies that restrict calories or carbohydrates have proven highly successful in the treatment of cancer both in combination with conventional therapies or on their own.[77]

Being obese increases the risk of cancer.[78] Yet, it is not excess body fat that encourages cancer growth, but rather the high blood sugar levels that nearly always accompany obesity. High blood sugar is a risk factor for cancer even when a person's weight or body mass index is normal.[79] Even mild elevations in blood glucose that would ordinarily be considered typical (fasting blood glucose between 95 and 108 mg/5.3-6.0 mmol/l) is associated with an elevated risk of cancer.[80] If you are concerned about the possibility of developing cancer, whether it be lung, breast, prostate cancer or whatever, one of the best things you can do to prevent it is cut out the sugar.

6

Metabolic Syndrome

METABOLIC SYNDROME AND CHRONIC DISEASE

A newly identified illness is running rampant across the world. It is the number one killer worldwide, yet many people have never heard of it. Chances are you will die from it. This deadly disease is called metabolic syndrome. Heart attacks and strokes are just two of the end results of this condition.

Although this disease has been around for a long time, it has only become a worldwide menace over the past few decades. It was initially identified as a growing health problem in the early 1980s and has now mushroomed into a global epidemic.

One of the reasons so many people are unfamiliar with metabolic syndrome is because it isn't usually cited as a cause of death or even as a disease, but rather as simply a risk factor for each. Yet, metabolic syndrome is essentially the underlying disorder that leads to the vast majority of chronic diseases and death worldwide.

Metabolic syndrome is defined as an association between a cluster of five metabolic disorders that commonly occur together and which greatly increase the risk of heart disease, diabetes, Alzheimer's, and other chronic degenerative diseases. The American Heart Association and the National Heart, Lung, and Blood Institute identify a person as having metabolic syndrome if he or she has any three or more of the following five conditions:

High fasting blood glucose:
Equal to or greater than 100 mg/dl (5.6 mmol/l)

Abdominal obesity:
Men—equal to or greater than 40 inches (102 cm)
Women—equal to or greater than 35 inches (88 cm)

High blood triglycerides:
Equal to or greater than 150 mg/dl (1.7 mmol/l)

Low HDL cholesterol:
Men—less than 40 mg/dl (1.03 mmol/l)
Women—less than 50 mg/dl (1.3 mmol/l)

High blood pressure:
Equal to or greater than 130/85 mm Hg

Metabolic syndrome is an indication that the body is seriously out of balance chemically, hormonally, and metabolically. It is associated with chronic low-grade inflammation and excessive oxidative stress. While metabolic syndrome is most commonly linked with heart disease, diabetes, and obesity, it also increases the risk of a multitude of chronic degenerative diseases, including the following:

Alzheimer's disease
amyotrophic lateral sclerosis (ALS)
arthritis
chronic fatigue syndrome
chronic obstructive pulmonary disease (COPD)
coronary artery disease
diabetes
dysmenorrhea
gallstones
GERD
glaucoma
fibromyalgia
hyperandrogenism
hypogonadism
hyperuricemia
infertility
inflammatory bowel disease (ulcerative colitis, Crohn's disease)
irregular periods
irritable bowel syndrome (IBS)
kidney disease

leaky gut syndrome
low immune function (increased susceptibility to infection)
macular degeneration
multiple sclerosis (MS)
non-alcoholic liver disease
obesity/overweight
Parkinson's disease
periodontal disease
polycystic ovary syndrome
psoriasis
psychiatric disorders/depression/anxiety
sleep apnea
thyroid dysfunction (hypothyroidism, hyperthyroidism)
vascular dementia
some forms of cancer

A person with metabolic syndrome is at greatly increased risk of developing any combination of the above chronic degenerative conditions. Those who have metabolic disorders generally experience multiple chronic health problems. For example, a person who has diabetes, may also suffer with Alzheimer's disease, vision problems, and hormonal imbalances, and die from a heart attack. A person with Parkinson's disease may also experience diabetes, arthritis, periodontal disease, kidney disease, and chronic constipation, and die of a stroke.

Many things can contribute to metabolic syndrome, including physical inactivity, aging, exposure to environmental toxins, medications and recreational drug use, smoking, and genetics, but diet is the primary factor. Metabolic syndrome is fundamentally a nutritional disease brought on by the overconsumption of sugar and refined carbohydrates, accompanied by a deficiency of good-quality fat, protein, and fresh produce. We know this because each of the five markers for metabolic syndrome is adversely affected by excessive sugar and refined starch consumption and can be improved by removing these products from the diet and replacing them with whole foods and healthy fats. A recent study that reviewed all available long-term randomized controlled studies on the treatment of metabolic syndrome concluded that refined carbohydrate restriction is the single most effective intervention for reducing all the features of the syndrome and should be the first approach in managing diabetes and heart disease, with benefits occurring independently of weight loss.[1] Indeed, all chromic degenerative diseases would improve with the replacement of sugar with healthier foods.

From the evidence, it appears that excessive consumption of sugar and refined starch, not fat or saturated fat, is at the heart of most every chronic, degenerative disease that troubles our society. It is no wonder why the sugar industry has worked so hard to distort the facts and confuse the medical community and general public about its dangers. If you want to age prematurely and suffer the last half of your life with chronic disease, it appears that consuming a high-sugar diet is the quickest way to get there.

In the following sections, we will take a closer look at each of five markers for metabolic syndrome.

INSULIN RESISTANCE

Insulin resistance is an essential underlying feature of metabolic syndrome.[2] It has always been a major defining condition of the syndrome. Some investigators originally used the term "insulin resistance syndrome" to describe it. They assumed that insulin resistance is always present with metabolic syndrome and required evidence of it for diagnosis.

Insulin resistance can generally be determined by measuring blood glucose levels while fasting. In normal, healthy individuals, fasting blood glucose levels should range from 65 to 90 mg/dl (3.6-5.0 mmol/l). As insulin resistance begins to develop, fasting blood sugar levels rise consistently above 90 mg/dl (5.0 mmol/l).

When fasting glucose reaches 100 mg/dl (5.6 mmol/l) or more, insulin resistance is advanced and is one of the markers for metabolic syndrome. At this point, a person is entering the beginning stages of diabetes, often referred to as prediabetes. Although 100 mg/dl (5.6 mmol/l) is used as the cutoff, this does not mean that a fasting glucose level of 99 gm/dl (5.5 mmol/l) is normal or safe. Fasting glucose levels between 91 and 99 gm/dl (5.1-5.5 mmol/l) are elevated and indicate the beginning stages of insulin resistance and an increased risk of degenerative disease. Full-blown diabetes is diagnosed when fasting blood sugar reaches 126 mg/dl (7 mmol/l) or greater; at this stage insulin resistance is severe and health risks become very serious. Uncontrolled diabetes can lead to a myriad of complications, such as mental deterioration, kidney failure, heart attack, stroke, blindness, nerve damage, digestive troubles, gum disease, and many other degenerative disorders.

Insulin resistance and type 2 diabetes are caused by the excessive consumption of sugar and refined carbohydrates and the lack of other, more nutritious, foods. It is the carbohydrate in the diet that affects blood sugar levels. Fats, proteins, and fiber have very little effect.

Insulin pulls glucose into the cells, it also triggers the conversion of glucose into fat and pulls fat into the fat cells. Insulin is a fat storage hormone. When insulin levels are elevated the body is in a state of fat production and storage. If the pancreas is working properly, high blood glucose levels are accompanied by high blood insulin levels. Therefore, a person who is

107

insulin resistant is continually in a metabolic state in which fat is being produced and stored. For this reason, essentially everyone who is obese is insulin resistant to some degree. Consuming refined carbohydrates raises blood glucose levels and intensifies insulin resistance, which promotes continued fat storage.

While all those who are obese are insulin resistant, not all people who are insulin resistant are obese or even overweight. In a state of insulin resistance the pancreas, which produces insulin, must work overtime to pump out large quantities of the hormone. Over time, this constant high demand for insulin takes its toll on the pancreas and it begins to wear out and insulin production declines. Diabetics who no longer can produce adequate insulin on their own must depend on regular insulin injections to control their blood sugar. Such people are usually of normal weight or even underweight.

A person can have normal fasting blood glucose levels and be at normal weight, yet still be insulin resistant. The reason fasting blood glucose levels can appear normal is because the pancreas is still functioning well enough to pump out massive amounts of insulin when blood sugar levels rise too high. This puts excessive strain on the pancreas, and while it is able to handle the load for a time, it won't be long before it begins to burn itself out. As the insulin producing cells wear out and die, less and less insulin is produced. Often, by this time the person has become diabetic, and in addition, may need regular insulin injections to manage blood sugar levels because medications alone are generally not enough.

Such a person may see their fasting blood sugar as normal and have only one or two other risk factors for metabolic syndrome and think they are in the clear—this produces a false sense of security. If your other risk factors indicate that you have metabolic syndrome or are even coming close, you are likely insulin resistant and your fasting blood glucose readings are not picking it up. In this case, you need to get another blood measurement, called the A1C test. This is a far more accurate test for blood sugar.

Fasting blood sugar measures the glucose levels at the time of testing. The A1C test provides an average measure over the previous 3 months. An A1C reading of 5.7 or below is considered normal, and a reading of 6.5 or above indicates diabetes. Regardless of your fasting blood sugar reading, if your A1C reading is over 5.7, you are insulin resistant and should consider this marker a positive indication for metabolic syndrome. For this reason, it is a good idea when you get your fasting blood test to also measure your A1C.

ABDOMINAL OBESITY

Obesity research has generally focused on the quantity of fat rather than on the distribution of fat on the body. However, where fat accumulates

108

can have a strong influence on health. In the 1940s Jean Vague, a French physician, observed that people with larger waists had a higher risk of premature cardiovascular disease and death than people who had slimmer waists or carried more of their excess weight around their hips and thighs. Over the next several decades this relationship continued to be observed. Studies found that not only the degree of obesity but also the location of body fat was a risk factor for diabetes, stroke, heart attack, and death from all causes. Waist circumference was a better predictor of cardiovascular disease and death than the degree of overweight.[3]

Abdominal (or upper-body) obesity results in an "apple-shaped" body, which is in contrast to a "pear-shaped" body, where excess fat tends to collect more on the lower half of the body (thighs, hips, and buttocks). People who have a large waist, whether they are overweight or not, are at a higher risk of health problems than those with a smaller waist.

The Nurses' Health Study, one of the largest and longest studies to date that has measured abdominal obesity, looked at the relationship between waist size and death from heart disease, cancer, or any cause in middle-aged women. At the start of the study, all 44,000 subjects were healthy and all of them measured their waist and hip size. After 16 years, women who had reported the highest waist sizes—35 inches or higher—had nearly double the risk of dying from heart disease, compared to women who had reported the lowest waist sizes (less than 28 inches). Women with the largest waists also had a high risk of death from cancer or any other cause, compared with women with the smallest waists. The risks increased steadily with every added inch around the waist.

The study found that even women at a normal weight with a BMI less than 25 were at a higher risk if they were carrying more of that weight around their waist: normal-weight women with a waist of 35 inches or larger had three times the risk of death from heart disease, compared to normal-weight women whose waists were smaller than 35 inches.[4]

It is recognized that some people who are not obese by conventional measures nevertheless are insulin resistant and may be diagnosed with metabolic syndrome. Although insulin resistant individuals need not be clinically obese, they nevertheless commonly have an abnormal fat distribution that is characterized by predominant upper body fat. Upper-body obesity correlates strongly with insulin resistance. Excess upper body fat can accumulate either abdominally (visceral fat) or subcutaneously (under the skin). Visceral fat is more strongly associated with insulin resistance than any other fatty tissue. A pattern of abdominal obesity correlates more strongly with insulin resistance and metabolic syndrome than does lower-body obesity.

Those people having a higher degree of insulin resistance can develop metabolic syndrome with only moderate excess in abdominal fat, but even

109

people with mild insulin resistance can develop metabolic syndrome if they accumulate marked abdominal obesity.[5]

The overconsumption of sugar, and particularly fructose and galactose, is the primary cause of abdominal obesity. Fructose and galactose are metabolized in the liver, where they are immediately converted into fat and glucose. When calories are plentiful, the liver converts these sugars mostly into fat rather than glucose. This is the fat that accumulates in the liver and around the organs as visceral or belly fat. In contrast to subcutaneous fat, visceral fat is very metabolically active. It releases fatty acids, inflammatory agents, and hormones that ultimately lead to higher LDL cholesterol, triglycerides, blood glucose, and blood pressure, and promotes insulin resistance.[6] Visceral fat releases a continuous stream of inflammatory agents that cause chronic inflammation. Inflammation interferes with glucose metabolism, leading to insulin resistance.[7-10] While glucose increases blood sugar levels and consequently the risk of insulin resistance, fructose and galactose have a much greater initiating effect on insulin resistance because they are converted into pro-inflammatory visceral fat. If you have a big belly (or even a bit of a stomach pooch) or insulin resistance, you can thank sugar, and especially high-fructose corn syrup for that.

In the United States and some other countries, the current measure for abdominal obesity that is part of the diagnosis for metabolic syndrome was established by a joint effort by the American Heart Association (AHA) and the National Heart, Lung, and Blood Institute (NHLB). Europeans tend to follow the International Diabetes Foundation (IDF) recommendations, which puts more emphasis on abdominal obesity for the definition of metabolic syndrome. The IDF's definition uses a waist circumference threshold of 94 cm or more for men and 80 cm or more for women. Because there is some ethnic variation in body type, Asians use another set of numbers for their definition of abdominal obesity. For Asian populations, except for Japan, the IDF has set a threshold of 90 cm or more in men and 80 cm or more in women; for Japanese they are 85 cm or more for men and 90 cm or more for women. For Asians living in the United States the lower waist circumferences, as defined by the IDF for these populations, are appropriate as one of the risk factors in defining metabolic syndrome.

The IDF criteria were based on the observation that some people manifest features of insulin resistance and metabolic syndrome with only moderate increases in waist circumference (between 94 and 101 cm in men or 80 and 87 cm in women). The IDF puts more emphasis on the significance of abdominal obesity in contributing to metabolic syndrome and requires abdominal obesity as one of the three factors in the definition of metabolic syndrome.

To correctly measure your waist circumference, do the following:
• Remove clothing from your waistline.
• Stand straight and place a tape measure around your middle, just above your hip bones and level with your belly button. Align the bottom edge of the measuring tape with the top of the hip bone.
• Make sure the tape measure is snug but not too tight and is horizontal around your waist.
• Read the measurement just after you exhale.

Belly fat cannot be reduced by doing abdominal exercises. This type of exercise will strengthen your abdominal muscles, but will not get rid of stored fat. Low-calorie dieting can work, but only if you do not consume sweetened foods or desserts, regardless of how few calories you eat. Eating sugar promotes belly fat and makes it very difficult to lose weight. It is ironic that many weight-loss products are sweetened with high-fructose corn syrup, probably because of the mistaken belief that since it does not affect blood glucose, as other sweeteners do, it is okay. Likewise, many diet products use low-fat milk and nonfat powdered milk, which are rich in galactose. In addition to reducing calorie intake, to successfully lose belly fat requires eliminating all sugars from the diet.

DYSLIPIDEMIA

Dyslipidemia is an abnormal amount of lipids (fat and cholesterol) in the blood. Two blood lipids that are used to diagnose metabolic syndrome are HDL cholesterol and triglycerides.

Most of the interest in detecting and treating heart disease over the past 60 years has focused on evaluating blood cholesterol values. The emphasis on cholesterol has been so great, almost to the exclusion of equally or even more significant risk factors, that high cholesterol has become synonymous with heart disease. Although elevated cholesterol is only a risk factor, most people believe it is more than that, and is the number one cause of heart disease.

A variety of blood lipid values are measured to evaluate heart disease risk, including total cholesterol, low-density lipoprotein (LDL cholesterol), high-density lipoprotein (HDL cholesterol), and triglycerides. Over the years, total cholesterol and LDL cholesterol have been emphasized the most to determine heart disease risk. And although still used, both have fallen out of favor among serious researchers and physicians. Total cholesterol in itself has proved to be nearly useless as a predictor of heart disease primarily because it lumps all forms of cholesterol into one value, including LDL (the so-called bad cholesterol) and HDL the good cholesterol, and

111

you don't know how much of each makes up the total. Researchers moved more toward measuring LDL cholesterol as a better indicator, but that has not been satisfactory either. We now know there are two types of LDL, one that is beneficial because it is essential for health, and the other potentially harmful because it is easily oxidized. That leaves HDL cholesterol and triglyceride values as the best common lipid indicators for heart disease risk.

HDL is considered protective against heart disease because it is believed to remove cholesterol from the arteries. Increasing HDL values lowers the risk of heart disease. Blood triglycerides are a measurement of fats carried by very low-density lipoproteins and are an independent risk factor for heart disease. High blood triglyceride values increase risk. For lowest risk, you want high HDL and low triglyceride values.

Many studies have shown that sugar consumption does just the opposite—it lowers HDL and raises blood triglycerides, thus increasing risk of heart disease. An example is a study published in the *Journal of the American Medical Association* (JAMA). The study examined sugar consumption and markers for cardiovascular disease of 6,113 adults who participated in the National Health and Nutrition Examination Survey (NHANES). The researchers investigated the effect of the consumption of added sugars on blood lipid levels.

The results showed that the greater the sugar consumption, the lower the HDL and the higher the triglyceride levels. High sugar consumption was also associated with an increase in the triglyceride/HDL ratio, which is a much more accurate measure of heart disease risk than either measure alone. Sugar intake also increased LDL levels, further reinforcing the detrimental effect sugar has on cardiovascular health.[11]

In another study, researchers at the University of California–Davis investigated what effects fructose, high-fructose corn syrup, and glucose had on blood levels of LDL cholesterol, triglycerides, and apolipoprotein-B (another cholesterol-related marker for heart disease risk). Using the 2010 *Dietary Guidelines for Americans* as their guide, the researchers used the maximum amount of sugar that was recommended as safe, which was 25 percent of total energy intake. It only took 2 weeks at this rate to significantly raise blood lipid levels, increasing the risk of heart disease. Fructose and high-fructose corn syrup had a greater detrimental effect than glucose.[12]

It makes sense that fructose would raise blood triglyceride levels more than glucose. Fructose is processed in the liver, where it is converted into glucose and fat (triglycerides). The fatty acids created during fructose metabolism accumulate as fat droplets in your liver and around your organs (visceral fat), causing insulin resistance and non-alcoholic fatty liver disease (NAFLD). Insulin resistance in turn progresses to metabolic syndrome and type 2 diabetes. The metabolism of fructose by your liver also creates a number of waste products and toxins, including a large amount of uric acid, which drives up blood pressure and causes gout.

HYPERTENSION

Hypertension is a chronic condition in which blood pressure in the arteries is persistently elevated. High blood pressure is called "the silent killer" because it usually has no obvious symptoms. However, over time, elevated blood pressure increases the risk for coronary artery disease, stroke, heart failure, peripheral vascular disease, vision loss, chronic kidney disease, and dementia.

Chronic elevated blood pressure is the most prevalent form of cardiovascular disease; in the United States it is believed to affect more than a third of the entire adult population. It contributes to half a million strokes and more than a million heart attacks each year. The higher the blood pressure is above normal, the greater the risk of heart disease. Hypertension is recognized as one of the major risk factors for heart disease.

A number of studies have investigated the association between the consumption of sugar in sweetened beverages and the risk of hypertension. The results have been mixed—a common problem in research when financial interests are at stake. To better understand the relationship between sugar consumption and high blood pressure, a team of international researchers gathered the most reliable studies on the topic and analyzed the data together. The combined meta-analysis included data on more than 700,000 subjects. The investigation confirmed the connection between sugar intake and high blood pressure with a pattern showing that the more sugar consumed, the higher the blood pressure.[13]

Dr. Richard Johnson, a professor of medicine at the University of Colorado, explains why sugar affects blood pressure in his book *The Sugar Fix*. "The primary culprit is fructose," he says. When fructose is metabolized it produces uric acid as a by-product. Uric acid is a normal waste product found in the blood; however, high levels are associated with gout, high blood pressure, overweight, and kidney disease.

Dr. Johnson has spent years studying the metabolic effects of fructose on animals and humans. At the University of Colorado he runs the kidney division and is in charge of transplantation and research on blood pressure. His interest in fructose wasn't aroused until he began to see a relationship between elevated uric acid levels and high blood pressure, kidney disease, and obesity. He discovered that 90 percent of obese adolescents newly diagnosed with high blood pressure also had elevated uric acid levels. He was able to normalize the blood pressure in 87 percent of these patients simply by lowering their uric acid levels.

113

It was known that purine-rich foods, such as beer, legumes, mushrooms, and fish, can raise uric acid, but that didn't explain the high levels in obese adolescents. There was something else in their diets that was having a greater effect on uric acid production, as well as promoting weight gain. It certainly wasn't eating a lot of fish and legumes. Dr. Johnson found the culprit to be high sugar consumption. Further investigation revealed that glucose didn't affect uric acid levels, but fructose had a major impact. When sucrose is consumed, the glucose fraction goes directly in the bloodstream; fructose, however, goes to the liver, where it is metabolized, producing uric acid as a by-product. In fact, fructose typically generates uric acid within minutes after ingestion. The consumption of high fructose corn syrup found in most processed foods supplies more fructose than white sugar, thus increasing the risk.

Before you begin thinking that the problem is only associated with fructose, it must be pointed out that glucose is not an innocent bystander. Glucose can intensify the effects of fructose and contribute its own detrimental effects on blood pressure.

Blood pressure is greatly influenced by the elasticity of the blood vessels. When the heart beats, it pumps blood; with this surge of blood, the arteries expand, allowing it to flow easily along its path through the body. If the blood vessels become stiff, they cannot expand easily. The heart has to work harder and blood pressure rises. This increase in force can cause minute rips and tears within the artery wall, followed by inflammation and leading to the development of atherosclerosis.

Dr. Michael Shechter and colleagues at Tel Aviv University in Israel have observed that high glycemic index foods that are rich in glucose rapidly increase blood pressure. This is not a new discovery, as doctors have known for decades that too much sugar and refined starch can be detrimental to cardiovascular health. But what they discovered was that high-glycemic foods, such as sugar, white bread, and cornflakes, reduce blood vessel elasticity, increasing blood pressure and cardiovascular risk. What was more surprising was the speed at which these foods can affect artery function. Differences can be observed almost immediately after eating sugary foods.

"Doctors know that high glycemic foods rapidly increase blood sugar," says Dr. Shechter. "Those who binge on these foods have a greater chance of sudden death from heart attack. Our research connects the dots, showing the link between diet and what's happening in real time in the arteries."

The researchers looked at four groups of subjects. One group ate cornflakes mixed with milk, the second group a pure sugar mixture, the third bran flakes, while the last group was given a placebo (water). Over four weeks, the researchers observed how each meal affected the subject's brachial artery. The test uses a cuff on the arm, like those used to measure blood pressure, which can visualize arterial function in real time.

The results were dramatic. Before any of the subjects ate, arterial function was essentially normal. After eating, the monitor showed enormous peaks, indicating arterial stress in the high glycemic index groups—the cornflakes and sugar groups. "We knew high glycemic foods were bad for the heart. Now we have a mechanism that shows how," says Dr. Shechter. "Foods like cornflakes, white bread, French fries, and sweetened soda all put undue stress on our arteries. We've explained for the first time how high glycemic carbs can affect the progression of heart disease."[14]

During the consumption of foods high in sugar, there appears to be a sudden dysfunction of the artery walls. While the effects are temporary, when the arteries are aggravated like this over time, elasticity is reduced, leading to elevated blood pressure, resulting in damage to the artery walls.

THE REAL CAUSE OF HEART DISEASE
The Primary Causes of Death

Nearly 75 percent of all deaths in the United States are attributed to just ten causes, with the top three of these accounting for over 50 percent of all deaths. Over the last 5 years, the main causes of death in the United States have remained fairly constant. Of the top ten causes of death in the United States, eight are associated with metabolic syndrome, namely: heart disease, cancer, chronic lower respiratory disease, stroke, Alzheimer's disease, diabetes, kidney disease, and suicide.

The Top 10 Causes of Death in the United States
1. Heart disease
2. Cancer
3. Chronic lower respiratory disease
4. Accidents
5. Stroke
6. Alzheimer's disease
7. Diabetes
8. Influenza and pneumonia
9. Kidney disease
10. Suicide

Source: *National Vital Statistics Reports* 66, no. 5 (November 27, 2017).

The ten leading causes of death worldwide are only slightly different, with six of them being associated with metabolic syndrome, namely: heart disease, stroke, chronic obstructive pulmonary disease, lung cancer, diabetes, and Alzheimer's/dementia.

The Top 10 Causes of Death Worldwide
1. Heart disease
2. Stroke
3. Lower respiratory infections
4. Chronic obstructive pulmonary disease
5. Lung cancer
6. Diabetes
7. Alzheimer's disease and dementia
8. Diarrhea (dehydration)
9. Tuberculosis
10. Road injury

Risk Factors for Heart Disease
After decades of research, the underlying cause of heart disease is still debated. However, researchers have identified several conditions or markers that are often associated with those who have heart disease. These are called risk factors. Not everyone who has heart disease has all of the recognized risk factors; some people have few or even none of them. Risk factors may not necessarily cause heart disease; however, they do make the disease more probable. The more risk factors a person has, the higher his or her chances of dying from a heart attack or stroke. The most commonly recognized risk factors are these:

age
gender (being male)
smoking
stress
physical inactivity
heredity
blood cholesterol level
blood triglyceride level
obesity and overweight
diabetes and prediabetes
blood uric acid level
hypertension
homocysteine levels
systemic inflammation
periodontal disease
unhealthy diet (too few vegetables and too much sugar)

The first six—age, gender, smoking, stress, lack of exercise, and heredity—are unrelated to diet. Some of them—age, gender, and heredity—we have no control over. The remaining ten—blood cholesterol and triglyceride levels, obesity, diabetes, blood uric acid level, hypertension, homocysteine levels, systemic inflammation, periodontal disease, and unhealthy diet—are all diet related, and we can influence them.

After reviewing this list of diet-related risk factors for heart disease, how many of them are adversely affected by sugar consumption? The answer is "all of them." As seen in the first part of this chapter and the previous two chapters, every single diet-related risk factor is strongly influenced by sugar. In fact, sugar is the only common or unifying element that ties them all together.

Fats, on the other hand, do not promote any of these risk factors. Even saturated fat, which gets the brunt of the blame for causing heart disease, is not associated with any of these risk factors. Some people may say that saturated fat increases total cholesterol, and some, but not all, saturated fats do tend to increase total cholesterol; however, total cholesterol is not a very good indicator of heart disease risk. That's why the cholesterol ratio and triglyceride levels are used instead by most doctors. In those cases where saturated fats do raise total cholesterol, the rise in cholesterol is due primarily to an increase in HDL—the good cholesterol that protects against heart disease. Consequently, the cholesterol ratio is either unchanged or lowered, thus reducing the risk of heart disease. When you look at the dietary related risk factors, it becomes obvious what truly causes heart disease—sugar.

No Association Between Heart Disease and Saturated Fat

In recent years there has been a growing body of evidence showing that there is no association between saturated fat consumption and heart disease. In contrast with decades-old nutritional advice, researchers at Cambridge University have found that giving up eating fatty meat, cream, or butter has no beneficial effect on reducing the incidence of heart disease. "It's not saturated fat that we should worry about" in our diets, said Dr. Rajiv Chowdhury, the lead author of the study and a cardiovascular epidemiologist in the department of public health and primary care at Cambridge University.

Dr. Chowdhury and his colleagues sought to evaluate the best evidence to date on the relationship between dietary fats and heart disease. They conducted a "meta-analysis" of 72 previously published studies involving more than 600,000 participants from 18 countries. The key finding was that saturated fat, whether measured in the diet or the bloodstream, showed no association with heart disease. However, the researchers did find a link between trans fats, produced when vegetables oils are hydrogenated. But they found no evidence of danger from saturated fat.

The primary criticism of saturated fat is that it increases LDL cholesterol, the kind that has been assumed to raise the risk for heart attacks. But the relationship between saturated fat and LDL is complex, says Dr. Chowdhury. In addition to raising LDL cholesterol, saturated fat also increases HDL cholesterol, which is known to protect against heart disease. Not all LDL cholesterol is bad. The LDL cholesterol that is raised by saturated fat is a subtype consisting of large, fluffy particles that are harmless and actually essential building blocks for vitamin D, the sex hormones, cell membranes, and nerve tissue. Saturated fat may increase total cholesterol, but it does so by increasing HDL and the large, fluffy LDL cholesterol, both of which are beneficial.

In contrast to the large, fluffy LDL is the smaller, dense LDL cholesterol, which is potentially far more dangerous. These smaller particles are easily damaged by oxidization and are more likely to cause inflammation and contribute to the buildup of artery-narrowing plaque. An LDL profile that consists mostly of these particles usually coincides with high triglycerides and low levels of HDL, both risk factors for heart attacks and stroke.

The smaller, artery-clogging particles are increased not by saturated fat, but by sugar, sugary foods, and an excess of carbohydrates, says Dr. Chowdhury. "It's the high carbohydrate or sugary diet that should be the focus of dietary guidelines. If anything is driving your LDL in a more adverse way, it's carbohydrates."[15]

For decades, dietary guidelines have focused on reducing total fat and saturated fat intake, based on the presumption that replacing saturated fat with carbohydrate and unsaturated fats will lower LDL cholesterol and should, therefore, reduce cardiovascular disease. However, we have been doing this for the past few decades without seeing any benefit; indeed, chronic diseases in general have increased.

More and more studies are revealing that it is not fat that promotes heart disease but carbohydrate, particularly sugar and refined starch. For example, researchers at the National Center for Cardiovascular Disease in Beijing combined the data from 15 studies with a total of 438,073 participants to determine the relationship between carbohydrate and cardiovascular disease. Their meta-analysis of these studies showed that high-glycemic carbohydrates were associated with an increased risk of coronary artery disease and stroke, with a linear dose-response relationship—the higher the refined carbohydrate consumption, the greater the risk of heart disease.[16]

Another study by a different group of researchers involving more than 135,000 subjects in 18 countries showed that as carbohydrate intake increased, so did the risk of death. Fat intake, however, showed just the opposite, demonstrating no relationship between heart disease and dietary fat.[17]

When you look at the evidence and ignore the marketing hype and deception from the sugar industry and its friends, it is easy to see that sugar, not fat, is the primary force behind the high rates of heart disease and the increasing rates of chronic degenerative diseases spreading throughout the world.

SUGAR SUBSTITUTES
Nonnutritive Sweeteners

Nonnutritive sweeteners are sugar substitutes that provide no calories, and therefore, have no nutrient value, but are many times sweeter than sugar (sucrose). Other terms used to describe them include low-calorie sweeteners, artificial sweeteners, zero-calorie sweeteners, and high-intensity sweeteners. The most common nonnutritive sweeteners allowed for use in foods by the FDA include aspartame, sucralose, saccharin, acesulfame-K, and stevia.

Nonnutritive sweeteners have long been recommended as healthier alternatives to sugar. When nonnutritive sweeteners first came on the market they seemed like a dream come true. They have no calories, so there is nothing to be converted into fat to increase body weight, and because they don't contain any actual sugar, they don't raise blood sugar levels—a major concern for diabetics. Nonnutritive sweeteners allowed weight-conscious individuals, diabetics, and others the freedom to eat the same sweet foods and beverages they always enjoyed without worry.

When nonnutritive sweeteners were introduced they were hailed as a partial solution to our growing obesity problem. Since their introduction the obesity problem has turned into a full-blown epidemic. Ironically, the so-called solution to the obesity problem has turned out to be one of the major contributors to it! A growing body of evidence is demonstrating that sugar substitutes are not only harmful but actually worse for our health than sugar.

According to a meta-analysis study published in the *Canadian Medical Association Journal*, individuals who routinely consume nonnutritive sweeteners have an increased risk for long-term weight gain, obesity, high blood pressure, and heart disease—symptoms associated with metabolic syndrome. Evidence also suggests nonnutritive sweeteners could have negative effects on metabolism, alter gut bacteria, and increase appetite (promoting increased calorie consumption).[18]

The study examined the data from 37 previous studies that tracked the cardiovascular and metabolic health of more than 400,000 people who used nonnutritive sweeteners. The people weren't losing weight, and the longer studies—which were observing the participants for up to 10 years—noted that they were instead gaining weight, and they were more likely to be obese, have high blood pressure, diabetes, heart disease, and other health issues compared to those who did not use nonnutritive sweeteners (e.g., those who used sugar). In other words, nonnutritive sweeteners had a greater adverse effect on health than sugar.

It appears that nonnutritive sweeteners, which are promoted as a means to help us lose weight and keep the weight off and to prevent diabetes, are actually doing just the opposite and may be fueling our obesity epidemic and contributing to the soaring rise of type 2 diabetes. In the 1990s less than 10 percent of the population used nonnutritive sweeteners. By 2008, more than 30 percent of Americans reported daily use of nonnutritive sweeteners; today that number has increased to over 50 percent.[19] Today, there are literally thousands of diet beverages and foods on the market. The increased use of nonnutritive sweeteners has added fuel to the dramatic rise in metabolic syndrome.

Why Sugar Substitutes Cause Weight Gain and Other Health Problems

The above study substantiates the results of a number of other recent studies.[20-22] According to an Australian study published in the journal *Cell Metabolism*, nonnutritive sweeteners can stimulate appetite, leading to increased calorie consumption of up to 30 percent, thus promoting weight gain and other metabolic problems.[23] But that is not all. The University of Sydney researchers found that the chronic consumption of nonnutritive sweeteners promoted hyperactivity, insomnia, glucose intolerance (insulin resistance), a more intense perception of sweetness, and an increase in appetite and in calories consumed.

"We found that inside the brain's reward centers, sweet sensation is integrated with energy content. When sweetness versus energy is out of balance for a period of time, the brain recalibrates and increases total calories consumed," says Associate Professor Greg Neely, a coauthor of the study.

The sweeteners essentially cause the brain to send a message that not enough energy has been consumed, triggering a kind of starvation response that makes food taste even better.

When ordinary sugar is eaten, dopamine is released in the brain and blood sugar levels rise, causing a secondary stimulation to produce dopamine. When eating nonnutritive sweeteners, dopamine produces the initial sensation of pleasure, but the second effect doesn't occur because sugar-free sweeteners do not increase blood sugar levels. As a result, the body sends signals requesting more food to compensate.

Another study, published in the *American Journal of Public Health*, found that people who were overweight or obese ate more when they drank nonnutritive sweetened diet beverages. This kind of drink was linked to increased energy intake ranging from 88 calories per day for overweight participants to 194 calories for obese participants.[24]

Studies have shown that it doesn't matter what type of nonnutritive sweetener is used, whether it be aspartame or stevia, the effects are essentially the same—weight gain and increased risk of diabetes and other metabolic problems.[25] It is the sweetness combined with the lack of corresponding calories, not the particular chemical makeup of the sweetener, that causes the problem. Therefore, any nonnutritive or zero-calorie sweetener will increase appetite and promote weight gain and all of its accompanying problems.

Nonnutritive Sweeteners Increase Risk of Diabetes in Just Two Weeks

A recent study has shown that nonnutritive sweeteners not only increase the risk of type 2 diabetes but can do so after just a few weeks of use.[26]

The researchers gave healthy volunteers nonnutritive sweeteners, sucralose or acesulfame-K, equal to that of drinking 1.5 liters of diet soda every day. Tests at the end of the two week study period revealed that the sweeteners altered the subjects' glucose metabolism, causing elevated blood glucose and insulin levels. The study found that just two weeks use of nonnutritive sweeteners was enough to cause changes in the volunteers' ability to properly manage their blood sugar, sending them in the direction toward diabetes.

This discovery is in line with earlier research that had found that nonnutritive sweeteners promote obesity and insulin resistance in animals as well as humans. In one study, using 7 volunteers, glucose intolerance was discovered in 4 of the subjects in fewer than 7 days.[27] It is becoming evident that nonnutritive sweeteners are worse than sugar.

Nonnutritive Sweeteners Alter Your Gut Microbiome

Low-calorie sweeteners are not only harmful to us but they are toxic to our gut bacteria as well. Animal and human research shows that all nonnutritive sweeteners cause DNA damage in, and interfere with the normal and healthy activity of, gut bacteria. A study published in the journal *Molecules* revealed that the six FDA approved sweeteners tested "had a toxic, stressing effect, making it difficult for gut microbes to grow and reproduce."[28] Ariel Kushmaro, PhD, professor of microbial biotechnology at Ben-Gurion University and lead author, said, "We are not claiming that it's toxic to human beings. We're claiming that it might be toxic to the gut bacteria, and by that, will influence us."

Kushmaro's group are not the only ones who have reported that nonnutritive sweeteners alter the gut microbiome—the population of bacteria that lives in the digestive tract. Researchers at the Weizmann Institute of

Science in Israel were the first to report that nonnutritive sweeteners alter the gut microbiome and in so doing contribute to our growing epidemic of diabetes and obesity. Nonnutritive sweeteners appear to disrupt the body's ability to regulate blood sugar, causing metabolic changes that can be a precursor to diabetes and obesity. These are "the very same conditions that we often aim to prevent" by consuming sweeteners instead of sugar, said Dr. Eran Elinav, an immunologist at the Weizmann Institute, and coauthor of the study.[29]

According to the study, anyone who uses nonnutritive sweeteners is at greater risk of developing diabetes and being overweight because of the type of bacteria inhabiting their gut. The scientists performed a multitude of experiments, on mice and humans, to back up their assertion that the sweeteners alter the microbiome.

According to the researchers, the different mix of microbes changes the metabolism of glucose, causing levels to rise higher after eating and to decline more slowly than they otherwise would. High blood glucose increases the rate of fat production and storage.

In the initial set of experiments, the scientists added saccharin, sucralose (Splenda), or aspartame to the drinking water of 10-week-old mice. Other mice drank plain water or water supplemented with glucose or with ordinary table sugar. After a week, there was little change in the mice that drank water or sugar water, but the group getting artificial sweeteners developed marked intolerance to glucose.

When the researchers treated the mice with antibiotics, killing the bacteria in the digestive system, the glucose intolerance went away.

To further test their hypothesis that the change in glucose metabolism was caused by a change in bacteria, they performed another series of experiments. They took intestinal bacteria from mice who had drunk saccharin-laced water and inserted them into the digestive tract of the mice that had never been exposed to any saccharin. Those mice developed the same glucose intolerance. And DNA sequencing showed that saccharin had markedly changed the variety of bacteria in the guts of the mice that consumed it.

Next, the researchers turned to a study they were conducting to track the effects of nutrition and gut bacteria on people's long-term health. In 381 nondiabetic participants in the study, the researchers found a correlation between the reported use of any kind of nonnutritive sweetener and signs of glucose intolerance. In addition, the gut bacteria of those who used artificial sweeteners were different from those who did not.

Finally, they recruited seven volunteers who normally did not use artificial sweeteners and over 6 days gave them the maximum amount of saccharin recommended as safe by the Food and Drug Administration. In four of the seven, blood-sugar levels were disrupted in the same way as in mice.

Further, when they injected the human participants' bacteria into the intestines of mice, the animals again developed glucose intolerance, suggesting that effect was the same in both mice and humans.

Dr. Elinav said he has changed his own behavior. "I've consumed very large amounts of coffee, and extensively used sweeteners, thinking like many other people that they are at least not harmful to me and perhaps even beneficial," he said. "Given the surprising results that we got in our study, I made a personal preference to stop using them."

Childhood Obesity Starts in the Womb

The adverse effects of nonnutritive sweeteners are even seen in the children of women who use these sweeteners during pregnancy. The incidence of childhood obesity has more than doubled in the last 30 years. One-third of children in developed countries are now overweight or obese. Part of this problem is due to children consuming foods and beverages sweetened with nonnutritive sweeteners. Another part of the problem comes from mothers consuming nonnutritive sweeteners during pregnancy, which greatly increases the risk of their children becoming obese.

In a study published in the *Journal of the American Medical Association Pediatrics*, researchers examined 3,033 mothers and their children. More than a quarter of the women consumed nonnutritive sweetened beverages during pregnancy. There was no association between nonnutritive sweetener use and weight at birth; however, after one year infants whose mothers consumed nonnutritive sweeteners were more likely to be overweight.[30] This effect was not due to maternal body mass index, diet quality, total energy intake, or other obesity risk factors. There was no association of increased risk of being overweight if the mother consumed sugar-sweetened beverages. The reason for the increased infant weight was attributed to the mother's consumption of zero-calorie sweeteners during pregnancy.

Zero-calorie sweeteners alter the gut microbiome, shifting the microbiota toward populations that tend to promote weight gain and metabolic disturbances. During delivery, whatever type of microbiota inhabit the mother's digestive tract and birth canal will be passed on to the infant. Therefore, the infant will acquire the type of bacteria that promotes weight gain, leading to weight problems later on.

As more evidence accumulates, it is becoming increasingly evident that nonnutritive sweeteners are causing more harm than good and are not suitable substitutes for sugar.

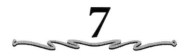

7

Understanding Fats

WHAT ARE FATS?
Lipids, Triglycerides, and Fatty Acids

The term *lipid* is often used when speaking about fat. *Lipid* is a general term that includes several fat-like or fat-soluble compounds in the body. By far the most abundant and the most important of the lipids are the triglycerides. When we speak of fats and oils we are usually referring to triglycerides. Two other lipids—phospholipids and sterols (which include cholesterol)—technically are not fats because they are not triglycerides. But they have similar characteristics and are often loosely referred to as fats.

The words *fat* and *oil* are often used interchangeably. Generally speaking, the only real difference is that fats are considered solid at room temperature while oils remain liquid. Lard, for example, would be referred to as a fat, while corn oil is called an oil. Both, however, are fats.

When you cut into a steak, the white fatty tissue you see is composed of triglycerides (cholesterol is also present on the cellular level and undetectable with the naked eye). The fat that is a nuisance to us, the type that hangs on our arms, looks like jelly on our thighs, and can make your stomach look like a spare tire, is composed of triglycerides. Triglycerides are not unique to humans and animals, but are found in plants as well. The bottle of corn or soybean oil in your kitchen cabinet is composed of triglycerides. It is the triglycerides that make up our body fat and the fat we see and eat in our foods. About 95 percent of the lipids in our diet, from both plant and animal sources, are triglycerides.

Triglycerides are composed of individual fat molecules known as *fatty acids*. It takes three fatty acid molecules to make a single triglyceride

COMPARISON OF DIETARY FATS

	Saturated Fats	Monounsaturated Fats	Polyunsaturated Fats
Safflower oil	9%	13%	78%
Grapeseed oil	7%	21%	72%
Sunflower oil	11%	20%	69%
Walnut oil	10%	24%	66%
Corn oil	13%	25%	62%
Soybean oil	15%	24%	61%
Cottonseed oil	27%	19%	54%
Sesame seed oil	15%	42%	43%
Peanut oil	18%	48%	34%
Canola oil	7%	62%	31%
Apricot kernel oil	6%	63%	31%
Chicken fat	31%	47%	22%
Almond oil	9%	73%	18%
Avacado oil	12%	74%	14%
Lard	41%	47%	12%
Palm oil	50%	40%	10%
Olive oil	14%	77%	9%
Macadamia nut oil	14%	79%	7%
Beef fat	52%	44%	4%
Butter/Ghee	66%	30%	4%
Palm kernel oil	82%	15%	3%
Coconut oil	92%	6%	2%

Saturated Fats   Monounsaturated Fats   Polyunsaturated Fats molecule. Fatty acids are linked together by a single glycerol molecule. The glycerol molecule acts as a backbone, so to speak, for the triglyceride.

There are dozens of different types of fatty acids. Scientists have grouped these into three general categories: saturated, monounsaturated, and polyunsaturated. Each category contains several members. So, there are many different types of saturated fat, just as there are many types of monounsaturated and polyunsaturated fats.

No dietary oil is composed purely of saturated, monounsaturated, or polyunsaturated fat. All natural fats and oils consist of a mixture of the three classes of fatty acids. To say an oil is saturated or monounsaturated is a gross oversimplification. Olive oil is often called "monounsaturated" because it is *predominantly* monounsaturated, but, like all vegetable oils, it also contains some polyunsaturated and saturated fat as well (see table below for the amounts of each kind of fatty acid found in different fats and oils).

Animal fats are generally the highest in saturated fat. Vegetable oils contain saturated fat as well as monounsaturated and polyunsaturated fat. Most vegetable oils are high in polyunsaturated fats, the exception being palm and coconut oils, which are very high in saturated fat. Coconut oil contains as much as 92 percent saturated fat—more than any other oil, including beef fat and lard.

There are many factors that contribute to the healthfulness of each type of fat—its saturation, the size of the carbon chain, and its susceptibility to peroxidation and free-radical generation.

Saturated and Unsaturated Fatty Acids

We hear the terms *saturated, monounsaturated,* and *polyunsaturated* all the time, but what do they mean? What is saturated fat saturated with?

Fatty acids consist almost entirely of two elements—carbon (C) and hydrogen (H). The carbon atoms are hooked together like links in a long chain. Attached to each carbon atom are two hydrogen atoms. In a saturated fatty acid, each carbon atom is attached to a pair of hydrogen atoms (see illustration below). In other words, it is "saturated with" or holding as many hydrogen atoms as it possibly can. Hydrogen atoms are always attached in pairs. If one pair of hydrogen atoms is missing, you would have a monoun-saturated fatty acid. "Mono" indicates one pair of hydrogen atoms is missing, while "unsaturated" indicates the fatty acid is not fully saturated with hydrogen atoms. If two, three, or more pairs of hydrogen atoms are missing, you have a polyunsaturated fatty acid ("poly" means "more than one").

Wherever a pair of hydrogen atoms is missing, the adjoining carbon atoms must form a double bond (see the illustrations opposite), which produces a weak link in the carbon chain that can have a dramatic influence on the stability of the fatty acid.

```
    H  H  H  H  H  H  H  H  H  H  H  H  H  H  H  H  H  H  O
    |  |  |  |  |  |  |  |  |  |  |  |  |  |  |  |  |  |  ‖
 H--C--C--C--C--C--C--C--C--C--C--C--C--C--C--C--C--C--C--O--H
    |  |  |  |  |  |  |  |  |  |  |  |  |  |  |  |  |  |
    H  H  H  H  H  H  H  H  H  H  H  H  H  H  H  H  H  H
```

Figure 1: Saturated fats are loaded, or saturated, with all the hydrogen (H) atoms they can carry. The example shown above is stearic acid, an 18-carbon saturated fat commonly found in beef fat.

```
    H  H  H  H  H  H  H  H        H  H  H  H  H  H  H  H  O
    |  |  |  |  |  |  |  |        |  |  |  |  |  |  |  |  ‖
 H--C--C--C--C--C--C--C--C--C=C--C--C--C--C--C--C--C--C--O--H
    |  |  |  |  |  |  |  |  |  |  |  |  |  |  |  |  |  |
    H  H  H  H  H  H  H  H  H  H  H  H  H  H  H  H  H  H
```

Figure 2: If one pair of hydrogen atoms is removed from the saturated fat, the carbon atoms would form double bonds with one another in order to satisfy their bonding requirements. The result would be an unsaturated fat. In this case it would form a monounsaturated fatty acid. The example shown is oleic acid, an 18-chain monounsaturated fatty acid that is found predominantly in olive oil.

```
    H  H  H  H  H        H        H  H  H  H  H  H  H  O
    |  |  |  |  |        |        |  |  |  |  |  |  |  ‖
 H--C--C--C--C--C--C=C--C--C=C--C--C--C--C--C--C--C--C--O--H
    |  |  |  |  |  |  |  |  |  |  |  |  |  |  |  |  |  |
    H  H  H  H  H  H  H  H  H  H  H  H  H  H  H  H  H
```

Figure 3: If two or more pairs of hydrogen atoms are missing and more than one double carbon bond is present, it is referred to as a polyunsaturated oil. The example illustrated is linoleic acid, an 18-chain polyunsaturated acid. This is the most common fatty acid in the majority of vegetable oils.

Short, Medium, and Long Chain Fatty Acids

The size or length of the fatty acid chain is also important. Some fatty acids contain only two carbon atoms, while others have as many as 24 or more. Acetic acid, found in vinegar, has a chain only two carbon atoms long. A longer acid chain may have four, six, eight, or more carbon atoms. Naturally occurring fatty acids most often occur in even numbers. Butyric acid, one type of fatty acid commonly found in butter, consists of a four-carbon chain. The predominant fatty acids found in meats and fish are 14 or more

127

carbon atoms long. Stearic acid, common in beef fat, has an 18-carbon chain. The 14- to 24-carbon fatty acids are known as long chain fatty acids (LCFAs). Medium chain fatty acids (MCFAs) range from 6 to 12 carbons, and short chain (SCFAs) are less than 6 carbons. The length of the carbon chain is a key factor in the way dietary fat is digested and metabolized and how it affects the body.

When three fatty acids of similar length are joined together by a glycerol molecule, the resulting molecule is referred to as a long chain triglyceride (LCT), medium chain triglyceride (MCT), or short chain triglyceride (SCT). You will often see *medium chain triglyceride* or *MCT* listed as an ingredient on food and supplement labels. To make things a little more complicated, you can also have triglycerides with the glycerol attached to a mixture of short, medium, or long fatty acids.

Both the degree of saturation and the length of the carbon chain of the fatty acids determine their chemical properties and their effects on our health. The more saturated the fat and the longer the chain, the harder the fat and the higher the melting point. Saturated fat, like that found in lard, is solid at room temperature. Polyunsaturated fat, like corn oil, is liquid at room temperature. Monounsaturated fat is liquid at room temperature, but in the refrigerator it becomes semisolid.

The table on the following page lists the most common fatty acids found in foods. The fats found in animal tissue, as well as our own bodies, are mainly the triglycerides consisting of stearic, palmitic, and oleic acids. Oleic acid is a monounsaturated fat. Stearic and palmitic acids are saturated fats. The saturated fats found in food consist of a mixture of the different types. Milk, for example contains palmitic, myristic, stearic, lauric, butyric, caproic, caprylic, and capric acids. Each of the fatty acids exerts different effects on the body that are governed by the length of the carbon chain and the degree of unsaturation (number of double bonds).

Saturated fatty acids with up to 26 carbon atoms (C:26) and as few as 2 carbons (C:2) in the chain have been identified as constituents of fats. Of these, palmitic acid (C:16) is the most common, occurring in almost all fats. Myristic (C:14) and stearic (C:18) acids are other common saturated fatty acids.

Short chain fatty acids (SCFAs) are relatively rare. The most common sources are vinegar and butter. Milk contains small amounts of the shorter chain fatty acids. These fats are concentrated in the making of butter and comprise about 4 percent of its total fat content. Medium chain fatty acids are also relatively rare but are most commonly found in some tropical seeds and oils, most notably, coconut.

Long chain fatty acids are by far the most abundant fatty acids found in nature. They provide the most efficient or compact energy package and

Carbons and Double Bonds in Fatty Acids

Fatty Acid	Carbons	Double Bonds	Common Source
Saturated Fatty Acids			
Acetic	2	0	Vinegar
Butyric	4	0	Butterfat
Caproic	6	0	Butterfat
Caprylic	8	0	Coconut oil
Capric	10	0	Coconut oil
Lauric	12	0	Coconut oil
Myristic	14	0	Nutmeg oil
Palmitic	16	0	Animal/vegetable oils
Stearic	18	0	Animal/vegetable oils
Arachidic	20	0	Peanut oil
Monounsaturated Fatty Acids			
Palmitoleic	16	1	Butterfat
Oleic	18	1	Olive oil
Erucic	22	1	Rapeseed oil
Polyunsaturated Fatty Acids			
Linoleic	18	2	Vegetable oils
Alpha-linolenic	18	3	Linseed oil
Arachidonic	20	4	Lecithin
Eicosapentaenoic	20	5	Fish oils
Docosahexaenoic	22	6	Fish oils

thus make the best storage fats in both plants and animals. Fat cells in our bodies and those of animals are almost entirely long chained, as are the fats in plants. The vast majority of the fats in our diet are composed of long chain fatty acids.

THE ESSENTIAL FATTY ACIDS
Polyunsaturated Fats

Polyunsaturated fats are found most abundantly in plants. Vegetables oils, such as soybean oil, safflower oil, sunflower oil, cottonseed oil, corn oil, and flaxseed oil, are composed predominantly of polyunsaturated fatty acids and, therefore, are commonly referred to as polyunsaturated oils.

Some fatty acids are classified as being essential. This means our bodies cannot make them from other nutrients, so we must have them in our diet in order to achieve and maintain good health. Our bodies can manufacture saturated and monounsaturated fats from other foods. However, we do not have the ability to manufacture polyunsaturated fats. Therefore, it is *essential* that they be included in our diet.

Two families of polyunsaturated fatty acids are important to human health: omega-6 and omega-3 polyunsaturated fatty acids. There are several omega-6 and omega-3 fatty acids. Two are considered essential because it is believed that the body can use these two to make all of the rest—linoleic acid and alpha-linolenic acid. These are the essential fatty acids (EFAs) nutritionists often talk about. Linoleic acid belongs to the omega-6 family. Alpha-linolenic acid belongs to the omega-3 family.

Theoretically, if you eat an adequate source of linoleic acid, the body can make all the other omega-6 fatty acids it needs. Likewise, if you have an adequate source of alpha-linolenic acid, it can make all the other omega-3 fatty acids.

Lauric acid, a medium chain saturated fatty acid, is considered conditionally essential—meaning it is essential at a certain stage in life. It, too, is not produced in the human body to any great extent, and therefore, must come from the diet. Infants need lauric acid for proper growth and development and to aid in establishing a healthy gut microbiome. Fortunately, mother's milk is a good source of lauric acid. In fact, all mammal milks contain lauric acid for the same reasons. In the event that an infant cannot breastfeed, commercial infant formulas all contain lauric acid to provide this essential nutrient. Two other medium chain saturated fatty acids, caprylic and capric acids, may also be conditionally essential, as they have much of the same effects as lauric acid and are also found in mother's milk. The richest dietary sources for all three of these medium chain fatty acids are coconut and palm kernel oils. While medium chain fatty acids are not considered essential for adults, they do serve many important functions that have a positive impact on health.

Linoleic and alpha-linolenic acids can be incorporated into cell membranes with other fatty acids or used as a source of energy; however, their most important function is as the precursors for the production of eicosanoids—hormone-like substances that participate in the regulation of inflammation, blood pressure, kidney function, cholesterol synthesis, and other physiological processes.

Fish, shellfish, free-range chickens, and animals that feed on grass and leafy foliage transform the linoleic and alpha-linolenic fatty acids in the algae and plants they eat into longer chain omega-3 and omega-6 fatty acids that are eventually converted into eicosanoids. Two long chain omega-3 fatty acids, eicosapentaenoic acid (EPA) and docosahexaenoic acid (DHA), are essential components of our brain and eyes.[1-2] A deficiency in these important fatty acids can seriously affect brain function and vision. Essential fatty acids are also necessary for healthy skin, hair, and mucous membranes. A deficiency can lead to numerous symptoms including dry and pale skin, scaly dermatitis, irregular or quilted appearance of the skin, thick or cracked calluses, weak or brittle fingernails, dry or brittle hair, hair loss, and dry eyes and mouth. Other symptoms include edema, kidney dysfunction, high blood pressure, numbness of the extremities, joint swelling, gastrointestinal distress, immune malfunction, raised cholesterol, and atherosclerosis.

In the human body alpha-linolenic acid is used primarily for the production of energy, as the conversion of this fatty acid to EPA and DHA is not very efficient. Human studies have shown that only 5 percent of the alpha-linolenic acid is converted into EPA and less than 0.5 percent is converted into DHA—the main essential fatty acid required for proper brain function.[3] Therefore, to satisfy our omega-3 requirements it is necessary to include in our diet animal-based foods rich in these long chain essential fatty acids.

EFA deficiencies are generally rare, being seen most often in studies with experimental or restricted diets, with improper infant feeding, as a symptom of malnutrition, or as a consequence of fad dieting. The popularity of low-fat diets, especially very low-fat diets, in recent years has greatly increased the number of people affected.

Nathan Pritikin, a self-proclaimed nutritionist, became famous in the 1970s and 1980s as one of America's leading advocates for low-fat dieting as a means of achieving optimal health. He founded the Pritikin Longevity Center to promote his low-fat program. Pritikin was a fanatic about keeping fat out of the diet. He claimed there was enough fat in lettuce and other vegetables to meet our body's needs. His diet limited fat consumption to a mere 10 percent of total calories. People lost weight, but they also developed health problems as a result of fat deficiency. In his book *Heart Frauds*, Charles T. McGee, MD, describes patients who came to him for treatment after they had been on the Pritikin low-fat diet. "Pritikin Program patients become deficient in essential fatty acids after they have been on the diet about two years," says Dr. McGee. "These people entered the office looking gaunt, with skin that was dry, droopy, pale, gray, and flaky (classic signs of EFA deficiency). Fortunately, this complication was seldom seen because most people find it difficult to keep fat intake down to the 10 percent level without cheating."

Pritikin claimed his low-fat way of eating would improve health, remove excess weight, and ward off degenerative disease. Unfortunately for Pritikin, it didn't work for him. He developed leukemia, went into deep depression, and committed suicide. Low immune function, depression, and suicide are well-known side effects of low-fat dieting.[4-5] Even diets that allow 25 percent of calories as fat, over twice that recommended by Pritikin, can seriously affect mental health.[6] The diet he advocated to achieve optimal health and increase longevity and happiness was the thing that drove him out of his mind and to an early death.

131

Another famous low-fat advocate was Roy L. Walford, MD, a professor of medicine at UCLA medical school. Walford was considered one of the world's leading experts on calorie restriction and longevity. Since the 1930s researchers have observed that the lifespan of animals could be extended up to 50 percent by restricting the total number of calories they ate. Walford believed human lifespan could be extended to 120 years on a calorie restricted diet. He wrote several books on the topic, including *The 120 Year Diet* and *The Anti-Aging Plan*. His plan was based on the concept of "calorie restriction with optimal nutrition," or what he termed "CRON." He claimed it would "retard the basic rate of aging in humans, greatly extending the period of youth and middle age; postpone the onset of such late-life diseases as heart disease, diabetes, and cancer; and even lower the overall susceptibility to disease at any age."

Restricting the number of calories consumed was central to Walford's program. Since fat contains more than twice as many calories as either carbohydrate or protein, fat was almost completely eliminated from his diet. Walford began eating this way when he was in his early 60s and fully expected to live to be a least 100. But things didn't work out the way he had planned. He developed amyotrophic lateral sclerosis (ALS)—an irreversible brain wasting disease, and died at the age of 79. The average lifespan for a white American male at the time was 78 years.[7] So after nearly 20 years of following a calorie-restricted, low-fat diet, he added the sum total of only one year to his life and suffered with crippling degenerative brain disease for his last several years of it. Instead of protecting him from degenerative disease, his low-fat diet was the thing that eventually did him in.

Calorie restriction with optimal nutrition may very well extend lifespan and forestall aging, but the problem with Walford's diet was that he did not understand the importance of fat and how necessary it is for optimal nutrition. Studies have shown that people eating low-fat diets have a higher rate of death due to degenerative disease than those with higher fat intake.[8] High-carbohydrate, low-fat diets are known to increase the risk of ALS, which eventually took the life of Dr. Walford.[9]

One of the classic symptoms of most all neurodegenerative diseases is chronic inflammation. Chronic inflammation is destructive. While anti-inflammatory drugs have been suggested as a possible answer, for the most part they have proven ineffective. In fact, some accelerate the rate of neurodegeneration. Researchers continue to search for new drugs. The answer, however, is already available, and it doesn't require any drugs. Inflammation can be lowered through diet. In a study conducted at the University of Connecticut, investigators found that a low-carb, high-fat diet does an admirable job of lowering runaway inflammation. They showed that a high-fat diet (59 percent of calories as fat) greatly *reduces* inflammation and is much more effective than a low-fat diet (24 percent fat).[10-11]

Since the body can make fat from carbohydrate, some people claim we don't need to have fat in our diet at all. They claim that the fat that is found naturally in grains and vegetables is adequate to fulfill our needs. This is a fatal mistake. People do die from fat malnutrition. The cause of death may be attributed to some chronic or infectious disease, like ALS, leukemia, or suicide, but the ultimate cause may be due to a fat deficiency. This was the case with Sergine and Joel Le Moaligou. After their baby daughter Louise became listless, the Moaligous frantically called an ambulance to their home 90 miles north of Paris. By the time paramedics arrived, baby Louise was dead.

Medical examiners noticed the baby was pale and thin. The 11-month-old child weighed only 12.5 pounds (5.7 kg); she should have weighed around 20 pounds (9kg). She was obviously malnourished. On closer examination they found she was suffering from severe malnutrition, which had apparently left her susceptible to infection. She died of a pneumonia-related illness.

The parents were shocked to learn of their daughter's nutritional deficiencies because she had been exclusively breastfed. Believing that breast milk provided the best nutrition for their daughter, they couldn't understand why she failed to thrive. The problem wasn't so much the breastfeeding but an issue with the milk her mother produced. The child's parents were both vegans and avoided consuming any animal products, as well as any added fat. As a consequence, the mother's milk was deficient in fat as well as several important nutrients. The mother's strict low-fat, vegan diet is what ultimately led to her daughter's death.

There has not been a minimum daily requirement established for either of the two EFAs. However, there are safe and adequate recommendations. These aren't minimums to prevent deficiency disease, but the amounts that appear to both prevent deficiency disease and yet not be too large to cause undesirable or toxic effects. The International Society for the Study of Fatty Acids and Lipids recommends an adequate amount of linoleic acid to be 2 percent of total calories, and a healthy amount of alpha-linolenic acid to be 0.7 percent.[12] Assuming a 2,000 calorie diet, that would equate to 4.4 grams of linoleic acid and 1.5 grams of alpha-linolenic acid. One teaspoon holds 5 grams, so combined it would amount to a little over 1 teaspoon. The current average consumption of linoleic acid by adult men in the United States is 16.0 g/day, and by adult women, 12.6 g/day.[13] There is no upper limit that is generally accepted, but linoleic acid levels over 10 percent have been reported to cause toxicity effects. In a 2,000 calorie diet that would equate to 22 grams.

Both the omega-3 and omega-6 fatty acids compete for the same enzymes in our bodies, for this reason, consuming too much of one can cause a deficiency in the other. For optimal health it is believed that we should be consuming a ratio of about 3:1 omega-6 to omega-3 fatty acids. The typical Western diet, however, is way out of balance in favor of omega-6 fatty acids, with a ratio as high as 20:1. Consequently, many people are omega-3 deficient. The primary omega-6 in our diet comes from linoleic acid, which is the dominant fatty acid found in most polyunsaturated vegetable oils. Linoleic acid is also found in meats, grains, legumes, nuts, seeds, and just about all the foods we eat. Processed foods are another major source of polyunsaturated vegetable oil. For this reason, it is a good idea to limit the amount of polyunsaturated vegetable oils we get in our diet.

Oils Rich in Omega-6 Linoleic Acid

canola	corn
cotton seed	grapeseed
peanut	safflower
sesame	soybean
sunflower	

Good Sources of Omega-3 Alpha-Linolenic Acid

chia seeds
flaxseed
leafy greens (brussels sprouts, spinach, chard, etc.)
seaweed
walnuts

Good Sources of EPA and DHA Omega-3 Fatty Acids

algal oil	egg yolks (free-range)
fish	grass-fed beef
perilla oil	shellfish

Sources of MCTs

butter	coconut/coconut oil
goat milk and butter	MCT oil (fractionated coconut oil)
palm kernel oil	

To balance the omega-6/omega-3 ratio, it is usually preferable to reduce the sources of excess omega-6 in the diet rather than consume increased amounts of omega-3 fatty acids. Consuming too much polyunsaturated fatty acids from any source can create new problems.

It is generally recognized that we do not get more than 10 percent of our daily calories from polyunsaturated fatty acids. One of the reasons for this is because these fatty acids are highly vulnerable to oxidation, even inside our bodies. To a great extent, the fats we eat are used to build body tissues; if we eat a lot of polyunsaturated fatty acids, we will have an increased amount of these fats in our bodies. The more polyunsaturated fatty acids we have in our bodies, the more likely they are to oxidize and produce destructive free radicals.

The best way to get your EFAs is in the same way as your ancestors did—from your foods! You do not need to eat processed vegetable oils to satisfy your daily EFA requirements. You can get all your EFAs from foods. This is by far the best way to get them because while they are still packaged in their original cellular containers, they are shielded from the damaging effects of oxygen and protected by naturally occurring antioxidants to keep them fresh.

Omega-6 essential polyunsaturated fatty acids are found in almost all plant and animal foods—meat, eggs, nuts, grains, legumes, and vegetables. Even animal fats contain enough omega-6 fatty acids to satisfy your EFA needs. Omega-6 fatty acids are so abundant in the diet that a deficiency isn't likely. Less common are the omega-3 polyunsaturated fatty acids. You can get all the omega-3 fatty acids you need by making sure you include some fish, free-range eggs, and leafy greens as a part of your weekly menu. Grass-fed beef and game meats also supply omega-3 fatty acids. Cattle that graze on grass, which is rich in omega-3s, incorporate these fats into their own tissues. Grain-fed beef, however, is a poor source of omega-3 fatty acids.

Essential Fatty Acid Toxicity

When it comes to EFAs, a little is good, but a lot is not. Many essential and indispensable nutrients including zinc, selenium, iron, and vitamins A and D, can become toxic if consumed in too large a dose. We need small amounts of them, but eating too much can cause problems. In contrast, other nutrients, are relatively harmless even in large amounts. Saturated and monounsaturated fats are of this type.

Polyunsaturated fats need to be consumed in balance with each other. This is referred to as the omega-6/omega-3 ratio. Both linoleic and alpha-linolenic acids use the same enzymes to be elongated and eventually converted into eicosanoids. A balance is needed to maintain homeostasis. For example, some eicosanoids (derived from linoleic acid) are pro-inflammatory, while others (derived from alpha-linolenic acid) are anti-inflammatory. We need the ability to instigate inflammation when necessary to fight off an infection and stimulate healing, but too much inflammation can cause tissue injury and prevent healing. Consequently, too much of one will cause a deficiency in the other.

While too much of either omega-6 or omega-3 fatty acids can lead to problems, it is linoleic acid that is the most problematic. Excessive amounts of linoleic acid have been tied to increased risk of nutrient/antioxidant deficiency, elevated inflammation, platelet aggregation, cancer, and omega-3 essential fatty acid deficiency.[14-17]

At the beginning of the 20th century, fat from animal sources dominated the diet throughout most of the world. In tropical regions coconut and palm oils were often the predominant fats consumed. Saturated and monounsaturated fats were the primary fats in the human diet throughout human history. Fish, livestock, and game provided much of the EFAs, particularly the long chain omega-3 fatty acids—EPA and DHA.

Although these sources contained only small quantities of the omega-6 linoleic acid, the level was apparently sufficient to prevent essential fatty acid deficiency. During the course of the 1900s, there was a twentyfold increase in the consumption of vegetable oils, markedly increasing the consumption of linoleic acid.[18] This occurred as a consequence of their increased availability though improved processing and extraction methods, as a perceived cheaper and healthier alternative to saturated fats, and from recommendations to consume these oils to lower blood cholesterol levels.

Ancel Keys was instrumental is this shift away from saturated fats toward vegetable oils and linoleic acid. His Seven Countries Study put the majority of the blame for the rising incidence of heart disease on saturated fat consumption, causing consumers to shy away from animal fats and tropical oils. Keys also performed dietary studies demonstrating that linoleic acid could lower total blood cholesterol levels, and promoted linoleic-rich vegetable oils as a means to reduce the risk of heart disease. He stated that a 10 percent increase in calories from linoleic acid would correspond to a 13 mg/dl (0.72 mmol/l) decrease in blood cholesterol.[19] Based on his studies, vegetable oils rich in linoleic acid as well as purified linoleic acid were the first drugs used by doctors for cholesterol lowering.

This reduction in cholesterol included a reduction in both LDL and HDL cholesterol, which in the late 1950s and early 1960s were not measured separately. Most doctors at the time were unaware there was more than one type of cholesterol. Interestingly, it was later discovered that the reduction in HDL by linoleic acid was significant and actually increased the cholesterol ratio (total cholesterol/HDL), thus increasing the risk of heart disease.

Later research found that lowering cholesterol with the use of linoleic acid does not reduce the risk of death from heart disease. In a recent meta-analysis combining the data from more than 530,000 participants and 76 studies, the results indicated that replacing saturated fats with polyunsaturated vegetable oils does not reduce the risk of heart disease.[20] An even more recently published study on 9,423 men and women who were living in care facilities and whose diet was carefully monitored, showed similar results. The researchers found that linoleic acid reduced blood cholesterol levels by 13.8 percent; however, there was a 22 percent increase in the risk of death for each 30 mg/dl (1.7 mmol/l) reduction in serum cholesterol. Lowering the patients' total cholesterol levels with polyunsaturated vegetable oils actually increased their risk of dying from heart disease.[21]

The consumption of omega-6 and omega-3 fatty acids has changed markedly over the past century. Animal fat consumption declined while vegetable oil consumption increased dramatically. Researchers at the US National Institutes of Health calculated the per capita consumption of food commodities and availability of essential fatty acids for each year from 1909 to 1999.[22] In 1909 soybean oil consumption in the United States was minuscule. After World War II soybean oil became more plentiful, and by 1969 consumption increased to about 3 kilograms per person per year, becoming the most consumed vegetable oil in the country. In the 1970s consumption dramatically increased, and by 1999 average consumption had increased to 12 kilograms per person per year. In contrast, in 1999 animal fats (butter, lard, and beef tallow) each averaged about 2 kilograms per person per year. During this time, linoleic acid consumption increased from 2.79 percent of calories to 7.21 percent. The availability of alpha-linolenic acid increased from 0.39 to 0.72 percent. This change shifted the ratio of linoleic acid to alpha-linolenic acid from 6.4 in 1909 to 10.0 in 1999.

Since these two fatty acids compete for the same enzymes in the process of elongation and eventual conversion into eicosanoids, the amount of EPA, DHA, and omega-3 derived eicosanoids produced has been reduced. The consumption of linoleic acid has tripled and the amount of alpha-linolenic acid has doubled, while the consumption of animal-based EPA and DHA has remained relatively unchanged. Despite the fact that the total amount of omega-3 fatty acids has increased, the greater increase in dietary linoleic acid (omega-6), decreased the total omega-3 fatty acid status of the body. The increase in linoleic acid, in essence, has increased the risk of omega-3 deficiency. The simple remedy is to reduce vegetable oil consumption.

MONUNSATURATED AND SATURATED FATS
The Other Essential Fats

Since polyunsaturated fatty acids are often referred to as the "essential" fatty acids, we tend to view them as the most important fats. However, monounsaturated and saturated fatty acids are equally important to our health, if not more so. In fact, monounsaturated and saturated fats are so important to our health that our bodies have been programmed to make them out of other nutrients. Getting an adequate amount of these fatty acids is too important to be left to chance. Our bodies need far more monounsaturated and saturated fatty acids than they do EFAs—about 10 times more. What it doesn't get directly from the diet, it tries to manufacture itself. While the body can manufacture saturated and monounsaturated fats, if dietary fat intake is very low, it cannot make enough on its own for optimal health. We still need them in our diet to avoid nutritional deficiencies.[23-24]

The foods that we eat provide the building blocks for our cells and tissues. This is true for the fats we consume as well. The fat in a healthy human body consists of about 45 percent saturated, 50 percent monounsaturated, and only about 5 percent polyunsaturated. That's right. Only about 5 percent of the fat in a healthy human body is polyunsaturated. Consequently, the body's need for polyunsaturated fat or EFAs is very small, while your need for monounsaturated and saturated fat is far greater.

For these reasons, the majority of the fats we eat should consist of monounsaturated and saturated fatty acids. These are the fats needed to build cell membranes, body tissues, and hormones, and if need be, to serve as a source of energy. Saturated fats also function somewhat like protective antioxidants, helping to prevent unsaturated fats from oxidizing.

If you have a good diet, rich in saturated fatty acids and antioxidant nutrients, the free radicals that normally occur as a part of daily living are quickly extinguished without causing much trouble. However, if you eat few fresh fruits and vegetables and an excessive amount of polyunsaturated vegetable oils, the generation of free radicals can overwhelm your antioxidant reserves, leading to vitamin deficiencies, premature aging, and other problems.

Good Sources of Monounsaturated and Saturated Fatty Acids with Limited Linoleic Acid

almond oil	animal fats
avocado oil	butter
coconut milk/cream	coconut oil
cream	ghee
macadamia nut oil	olive oil
palm kernel oil	palm oil

Saturated Fat Does Not Promote Heart Disease

Probably no food component in history has been as misunderstood and maligned as saturated fat. It is labeled the cause of nearly every health problem of modern civilization. If it really is as dangerous as they say, it's

138

truly a miracle how our ancestors survived for thousands of years eating a diet dominated by saturated fat. Animal fats, butter, and palm and coconut oils were the most common fats used throughout history. Interestingly enough, when people ate primarily saturated fats, the so-called diseases of modern civilization—heart disease, diabetes, and the like—were uncommon. As we've replaced saturated fats with more sugar, refined carbohydrates, and polyunsaturated oils, these diseases have come upon us like a plague. From a historical point of view it is easy to see that saturated fats don't cause these diseases.

Rather than being a poison, as it is often depicted, saturated fat is a vital nutrient. It is necessary for obtaining and maintaining good health. Saturated fat serves as an important source of energy for the body and aids in the absorption of vitamins and minerals. As a food ingredient, fat helps us feel full and provides taste, consistency, and stability. Saturated fat is necessary for proper growth, repair, and maintenance of body tissues. It is essential for good lung function and is the preferred source of energy for the heart.

Over the years, many studies have sought to prove the cholesterol hypothesis of heart disease—that diets high in saturated fat and cholesterol promote heart disease. Results of these studies have been mixed. Some seemed to support it, while others did not. However, the majority of the medical community, along with the sugar and pharmaceutical industries (which profit greatly from the saturated fat-heart disease idea) support the theory. Those studies that appear to support the theory are heavily promoted by the sugar and pharmaceutical industries and, consequently, receive national press and are used as justification to establish government policies on health. Those studies that do not support the theory, however, have no big industry to publicize them and are generally ignored and forgotten.

The evidence in favor of the cholesterol hypothesis is no greater than the evidence that contradicts it. In fact, there is a substantial amount of evidence that challenges the hypothesis.[25] The number of studies for or against is not a major issue; some of the studies have used relatively few participants, while others have used much larger numbers. Obviously, the results of a study involving 50,000 test subjects carries more weight than one involving only 1,000. One large study using 50,000 participants produces more reliable results than 10 small studies with a total combined number of 10,000 participants. So, the total number of studies is not as important as the number of people *in* the studies. If *all* the subjects in these many different studies were combined and evaluated equally, what would the final outcome be? Would it prove the cholesterol hypothesis or disprove it?

Researchers at the Children's Hospital Oakland Research Institute in California set out to find the answer. They analyzed all the previous studies with data for dietary saturated fat intakes and risk of cardiovascular disease.

The studies also had to be of high quality and reliable. Twenty-one studies were identified that fit their criteria. This meta-analysis study included data on nearly 350,000 subjects. With such a large subject database, the results would be far more reliable than a study consisting of only 10,000 or even 100,000 subjects. The focus of the researchers was to determine if there was sufficient evidence linking saturated fat consumption to cardiovascular disease. Their results said no. Intake of saturated fat was not associated with an increased risk of cardiovascular disease. Those people who ate the greatest amount of saturated fat were no more likely to suffer a heart attack or stroke than those who ate the least. No matter how much saturated fat one ate, the incidence of heart disease was not affected.[26] This study demonstrates that the combined data from all available studies in the medical literature disprove the cholesterol hypothesis. Since the publication of this study in 2010, many other studies have been published that have confirmed these results—saturated fat consumption does not promote heart disease.[27-28]

A recent major study conducted by a team of international investigators evaluated the associations between fat and carbohydrate intake with cardiovascular disease and overall mortality in 18 countries.[29] The study included 135,335 individuals with a medium follow-up of 7.4 years. The study revealed that the risk of death increases as carbohydrate consumption increases. Intake of total fat, saturated fat, and monounsaturated fat was associated with a reduced risk of death. In other words, total fat, saturated fat, and monounsaturated fat intake had a protective effect against all causes of mortality. Polyunsaturated fats had a neutral effect—neither protective nor causative. Saturated fat consumption showed a pronounced protective effect against stroke. This study provided further proof that fats, including saturated fats, do not cause heart disease. It also showed that a diet high in carbohydrate increases the risk of death from all causes. The 37 researchers involved in the study concluded that dietary fat intake was not associated with cardiovascular disease and that the current guidelines by WHO, AHA, and other organizations recommending limits on fat and saturated fat intake were unfounded, and removing the current restrictions on fat intake and limiting carbohydrate intake would improve overall health.

NOT ALL FATS ARE HEALTHY
Oxidized Vegetable Oils
Some of the primary sources of fat in our diet come from restaurant and processed foods. Most of the fats we get from these sources are unhealthy. To make matters worse, at home we often damage oils during food preparation, causing them to lose their health benefits and even produce harmful by-products.

Unsaturated fats and particularly, polyunsaturated fats, are highly vulnerable to oxidation. When oxygen reacts normally with a compound, the compound becomes "oxidized." Unsaturated fats oxidize in a process that biochemists call *lipid peroxidation*. "Peroxidation" signifies an oxidation process involving fats that produce peroxide free radicals.

When unsaturated oils are exposed to heat, light, or oxygen, they begin to oxidize and form destructive free radicals. Once they are formed, free radicals can attack other unsaturated fatty acids and proteins, causing them to become oxidized and generate more free radicals. It is a self-perpetuating process.

Most cooks recommend polyunsaturated vegetable oils in cooking and food preparation as a "healthy" alternative to saturated fats. Ironically, these unsaturated vegetable oils, when used in cooking, form a variety of toxic compounds that are far more damaging to health than any saturated fat could be. Polyunsaturated vegetable oils are the least suitable for cooking.[30] The temperatures used in ordinary cooking accelerate the oxidation process. The higher the temperature and the longer the exposure, the greater the oxidation. The vegetable oils used in restaurants and food processing undergo high temperatures. Oils in deep fryers are often used continually for weeks without being replaced, causing them to accumulate high levels of free-radical by-products.

Polyunsaturated fatty acids are easily transformed into harmful lipid peroxides. Monounsaturated fatty acids are chemically more stable and can withstand higher temperatures, yet they too can oxidize and form toxic by-products if heated to high temperatures. Saturated fatty acids are very heat stable and can withstand relatively high temperatures with much less oxidation. All fats and oils contain varying mixtures of polyunsaturated, monounsaturated, and saturated fatty acids. Therefore, they all respond a little differently to exposure to heat. Polyunsaturated vegetable oils generally contain the highest amount of polyunsaturated fatty acids, and therefore, are the most vulnerable to lipid peroxidation. As monounsaturated and saturated fatty acid content increases, the oil becomes more heat stable. From the fatty acid composition (see the table at the beginning of this chapter), you can see that olive oil is more heat stable than corn oil, and lard is more stable than olive oil. Coconut oil, with a saturated fatty acid content of 92 percent, is more stable than all of them.

Martin Grootveld, PhD, a professor of bioanalytical chemistry and chemical pathology at De Montfort University in Leicester, has carried out a series of experiments on lipid peroxidation. He has found that a typical meal of fish and chips fried in vegetable oil, contains as much as 100 to 200 times more toxic oxidized by-products than the safe daily limit set by the World Health Organization. In contrast, heating up butter, olive oil, or lard in tests produced much lower levels. Coconut oil produced the lowest levels.

"For decades, the authorities have been warning us how bad butter and lard was," says Grootveld. "But we have found butter is very, very good for frying purposes and so is lard. People have been telling us how healthy polyunsaturates are in corn oil and sunflower oil, but when you start messing around with them, subjecting them to high amounts of energy in the frying pan or the oven, they undergo a complex series of chemical reaction which results in the accumulation of large amounts of toxic compounds." His recommendation is to avoid eating foods cooked in polyunsaturated oils.[31]

Therefore, saturated fats are the safest to use for day-to-day cooking and baking. The higher the temperature and the longer the exposure, the greater the number of lipid peroxides produced. The higher the polyunsaturated fatty acid content of the oil, the more vulnerable it is to oxidation.

Use saturated fats, like lard and palm oil, for medium- to high-heat cooking; monounsaturated oils, like olive oil, for low-temperature cooking and salads; and polyunsaturated oils for non-cooking purposes, or better yet, don't use them at all. Never cook or bake at any temperature using polyunsaturated vegetable oils, and avoid all restaurant and commercially processed foods containing them.

Hydrogenated Vegetable Oils

Many packaged foods are made using partially hydrogenated vegetable oil. These are among the most health-damaging fats you can possibly eat—just as bad, if not worse, than oxidized polyunsaturated fats.

Hydrogenation is a process in which polyunsaturated vegetable oil is chemically altered to form a more saturated fat. Increasing the saturation makes the oil less susceptible to spoilage and is cheaper than using animal fats or tropical oils. Hydrogenation involves heating vegetable oils to high temperatures while bombarding them with hydrogen atoms in the presence of a nickel catalyst. In the process, however, a new type of fatty acid, known as a *trans fatty acid*, is created. Trans fatty acids are man-made fats. These artificial fats are structurally different from natural fats. Our bodies can handle natural fats, but trans fatty acids have no place in our bodies and are linked to many health problems. Shortening and margarine are two hydrogenated oils that should be completely eliminated from your diet.

"These are probably the most toxic fats ever known," says Walter Willett, MD, professor of epidemiology and nutrition at Harvard School of Public Health.[32] Studies show that trans fatty acids can contribute to atherosclerosis and heart disease. Trans fatty acids increase blood LDL and lower the HDL, both regarded to be undesirable changes.[33] Researchers now believe they have a greater influence on the risk of cardiovascular disease than any other dietary fat.[34]

142

Trans fatty acids affect more than just our cardiovascular health. They have been linked to a variety of adverse health effects, including cancer, multiple sclerosis, diverticulitis, diabetes, and other degenerative conditions.[35] Trans fatty acids disrupt brain communication. Studies show that the trans fatty acids we eat get incorporated into brain cell membranes, including the myelin sheath that insulates neurons. Trans fatty acids alter the electrical activity of brain cells, causing cellular degeneration and diminished mental performance.[36]

Under pressure from many health organizations and the public, the United States Institute of Medicine spent three years reviewing all the published studies on trans fatty acids. After the study was completed, the Institute of Medicine issued a statement declaring that no level of trans fatty acid consumption was safe. What surprised everyone was that the Institute of Medicine didn't give a recommendation as to what percentage of trans fats were safe to consume, as is often done with food additives, but flatly stated that *no level* of trans fats is safe. If you see a packaged food that contains hydrogenated oil, margarine, or shortening, don't touch it. If you eat out, ask the restaurant manager what type of oil they use to cook their food. If they say vegetable oil, it almost definitely is hydrogenated vegetable oil: avoid it. The reason you can safely count on it being hydrogenated vegetable oil is because regular vegetable oil breaks down too quickly and becomes rancid. Restaurants like to reuse their oils as long as possible before they have to be tossed out. Ordinary vegetable oils have too short a lifespan.

Many of the foods you buy in the store and in restaurants are prepared with or cooked in hydrogenated oil. Fried foods sold in grocery stores and restaurants are usually cooked in hydrogenated oil because it makes foods crispy and is more resistant to spoilage than ordinary vegetable oils. Many frozen processed foods are cooked or prepared in hydrogenated oils. Hydrogenated oils are used in making french fries, biscuits, cookies, crackers, chips, frozen pies, pizzas, peanut butter, cake frosting, and ice cream, especially soft serve ice cream.

The World Health Organization (WHO) has been advocating the complete global elimination of hydrogenated oils. Some countries, such as Denmark, Switzerland, and the United States, have taken steps to ban trans fatty acids from their countries. The US Food and Drug Administration mandated the labeling of artificial trans fats on food products and the eventual elimination of them from the food supply. Food companies are gradually removing these dangerous fats from their products. While steps are being taken to reduce our exposure to trans fatty acids, it will likely be some time before all countries and food manufacturers are compliant.

8

Fat Is A Superfood

FAT IS GOOD FOR YOU

Some foods are called "superfoods" because they are loaded with vitamins, minerals, antioxidants, and other important nutrients and have been shown to help prevent, and in some cases even reverse, various health problems. These foods are heavily promoted as those that should be included in a healthy diet. Some that are getting a lot of attention are kale, blueberries, beets, seaweed, turmeric, goji berries, and noni juice. As good as these may be, there is one food that is not ordinarily included in the list that is probably the most powerful superfood of them all, and that is fat.

Fat can provide more nutrition, more benefit, and more protection against disease than the most acclaimed superfoods. If fat were some exotic vegetable or herb, it would be proclaimed from the housetops as a wonder food with multiple health benefits. The medical community would praise it for its nutritional and medicinal value. It would become the most popular superfood of all time.

Unfortunately, due to the efforts of the sugar industry and general misconceptions, fat has been vilified as the primary cause of our bulging bellies, thunderous thighs, and pudgy posteriors, not to mention the driving force behind our heart disease epidemic. Dietary fat, and particularly saturated fat, is blamed for contributing to just about every health problem experienced by mankind. Many people consider it nothing but a poison. To them it is an ugly beast lurking in our foods solely to do us harm, and we would be far better off eliminating all traces of it from our diet.

Eliminating fat from our diet would be a disaster: dietary fat is an essential nutrient that is required for us to achieve and maintain good health.

144

In fact, we couldn't live without it. It is far more important than carbohydrate, which makes up the bulk of most people's diets. You can live a long, healthy life without any carbohydrate, but you cannot live without fat. The sole purpose of carbohydrate is to provide us with energy. Fats can do that too, but in addition, they do a whole lot more.

Simply put, fat is good for you. It nourishes the body and can help protect you from disease. Contrary to popular opinion, fats don't cause disease, they help protect against it. It is surprising to most people how important fat is to our overall health. Let's look at some of the ways fats support good health and can rightly be called a superfood.

ENERGY SOURCE

Fat is fuel. Gasoline powers our cars; fat powers our bodies. Fat is one of the three energy-producing nutrients. The other two are protein and carbohydrate. Our bodies use fat as a source of energy to power metabolic processes and maintain life. About 60 percent of the body's energy needs are supplied by fat.

Every cell in our bodies must have a continual source of energy to function properly and maintain life. The body's first choice of fuel is carbohydrate. When there is adequate carbohydrate in the diet to meet energy needs, fat is put into storage inside fat cells. Excess carbohydrate and protein are converted into fat and also packed away into fat cells for use later. Between meals or during times of low food intake, fat is pulled out of storage and used to supply the body's ongoing energy needs.

Fat has more calories per gram than either carbohydrate or protein because it is a compact energy source that can be stored away and used later. Energy is measured in terms of calories. The body can store more calories as fat than it can as carbohydrate or protein. If the body stored protein instead of fat, you would look like a bloated pork sausage because your storage cells would double in size. So be thankful you store fat and not protein.

If you didn't have fat or adequate amounts of fat stored in fat cells, between meals and during prolonged periods of fasting, your body would resort to using protein, such as muscle tissue, for energy. Your body would literally consume itself to get the energy it needs to stay alive.

BUILDING BLOCKS

People tend to think of the fat in our bodies as just excess baggage hanging around our bellies and thighs, with no useful purpose. However, fat is found in more places than just our fat cells. Fat comprises a major structural component of our entire body. We may think of our bodies as being made primarily of water and protein, but fat comprises a major portion of our cells and tissues.

Fatty acids make up a major structural component of every cell in your body. The cells of your heart, lungs, kidneys, liver, and every other organ are dependent on fat to hold them together. Fatty acids are the dominant component of the cell membrane—the skin that holds the cells together. The organelles—the tiny cellular organs within the cells—such as the nucleus and mitochondria, are also encased in a fatty membrane.

Cell membranes envelop the organelles and cytosol (fluid inside the cell) and keep them separate from the fluids, chemicals, proteins, microorganisms, and other substances outside the cell. This membrane regulates which substances enter and exit the cell. For example, it can block the entrance of bacteria but allow oxygen and glucose to enter and carbon dioxide to exit. It also contains receptors for hormones that control cell activity.

The cell membrane is composed of a double layer of fat molecules called *phospholipids* embedded with protein and cholesterol. Phospholipids are similar to triglycerides in that they are composed of fatty acids attached to a glycerol molecule. However, the phospholipid only has two fatty acids; in place of the third fatty acid is a phosphate and nitrogen compound. There are many types of phospholipids, just as there are triglycerides, depending on the nitrogen compound and type of fatty acids they contain. Two that have gained some degree of interest are *phosphatidylcholine* and *phosphatidylserine*, both of which are essential for proper brain and digestive function. Studies have shown that as dietary supplements they might be useful in the treatment of dementia, depression, gallstones, liver disorders,

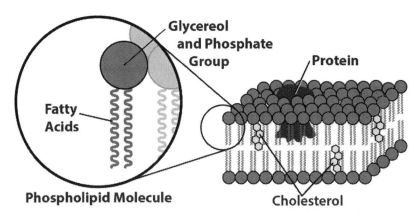

The cell wall is composed primarily of phospholipids arranged in a double layer.

146

and ulcerative colitis, and to counter the adverse side effects of nonsteroidal anti-inflammatory drugs.[1-4]

The biggest benefit appears to be with brain health. Nerve function depends on a high percentage of fat, and for this reason the brain is composed of 60 percent fat and cholesterol. To put it bluntly, a healthy, intelligent brain is full of fat.

Dietary fats are used not only to make structural components of cells, but also to make cholesterol, hormones, and prostaglandins that control and regulate bodily functions. Vitamin D, estrogen, progesterone, testosterone, DHEA, and many other hormones are constructed out of cholesterol. Cholesterol is essential for cell membrane integrity and aids in cell communication and function.

CHEMICAL MESSENGERS

Fatty acids supply the basic building blocks for our hormones—special chemical messengers in the body that control most major bodily functions. Hormones play a critical role in our body's chemistry and physiology. They affect our body's functions from growth and sexual development and mood to how well we sleep, how we manage stress, and how our body breaks down and processes food.

Hormones maintain homeostasis—a state in which the body is in balance chemically and physiologically. A lack of adequate fat in the diet can adversely affect homeostasis. For example, sexual development and function can be retarded or altered. Mental function, mood, hunger and appetite, and more can all be affected.

Fats don't just supply the raw material for building hormones, but can have hormone-like effects themselves. The most notable are the essential fatty acids. Polyunsaturated fatty acids can be transformed into signaling molecules called *eicosanoids*. Subcategories of the eicosanoid family include prostaglandins, prostacyclins, leukotrienes, and thromboxanes. The synthesis of eicosanoids involves a series of steps controlled by special enzymes. These enzymes cause oxidation reactions to take place in just one particular way to make a particular type of eicosanoid. These eicosanoids typically are not stored within cells but are synthesized as needed.

Eicosanoids exert a pronounced effect on how our bodies function and, for this reason, are very important. They are involved in the regulation of immune function, blood pressure, inflammation, cholesterol synthesis, platelet aggregation (clotting ability), cell growth, pain perception, and mucus secretion, to mention a few. Because eicosanoids affect so many vital functions of the body, the lack of adequate dietary fat can have far-reaching health consequences.

While saturated and monounsaturated fatty acids are not used in the production of eicosanoids, they can still exert hormone-like effects. Fatty acid receptors are found throughout the body, most notably the intestines, pancreas, and brain. These receptors are activated by specific fatty acids, which trigger a hormone-like response. These receptors are called G protein-coupled receptors or GPR. About 250 of these receptors are known and others are believed to yet be discovered. Each receptor is identified by a number. GPR41 and GPR43, which are located in the digestive tract, are activated by short chain fatty acids. GPR84 is a receptor for medium chain fatty acids, GPR40 for long chain fatty acids, and GPR120 is activated by omega-3 fatty acids, and so forth. Ketone bodies, which are derived primarily from stored body fat, are known to activate GPR41.[5] GPRs are involved in the regulation of gut hormones and digestive function, immune function, inflammation response, insulin secretion and sensitivity, sympathetic nervous system activity, and many other aspects of metabolic homeostasis.

Contrary to common misperception, dietary fats are not just sources of calories, but participate in the regulation of many critical physiological functions and are necessary to maintain homeostasis and enjoy good health.

WEIGHT MANAGEMENT

One of the reasons that people are overweight or have trouble losing weight is that they don't eat enough fat. Believe it or not, dietary fat can be a weight loss aid when it replaces carbohydrates in the diet.

Most of the fat in our bodies does not come from the fat in our diets, it comes from the carbohydrates we eat. All of the carbohydrate in our diet, which is not used immediately for energy, is converted into fat and stored in our fat cells. The vast majority of food we eat comes from carbohydrates. On average, we consume about 60 percent of our daily calories in the form of carbohydrate, only about 40 percent comes from protein and fat. Most of the protein and fat we consume is used as structural materials to build and maintain muscles, bones, and other tissues. Ordinarily, only a small fraction of the protein and fat we eat is used to produce energy or is stored as fat. The body does not need to use protein and fat in our diet for energy because there is so much carbohydrate available, even an excess. This excess carbohydrate is what ends up as body fat.

Studies have shown that a carbohydrate-rich diet, like we normally eat, increases the synthesis of fat and cholesterol. When some of the carbohydrate is replaced by fat, fat and cholesterol production in the body decreases![6] These studies disprove the theory that all calories are equal. Therefore, replacing most of the carbohydrate in the diet with fat will lead to less fat production and lower body weight (and cholesterol levels improve too). It is really that simple.

A series of interesting studies were conducted by researchers at the University of London. They investigated the relative effects of fat, protein, and carbohydrate on weight loss in a low-calorie diet. They put 14 obese patients on four different diets in succession over a period of time. Each of the diets provided 1,000 calories per day, but differed in the amount of fat, protein, and carbohydrate. One diet had 90 percent fat, the next 90 percent protein, the next 90 percent carbohydrate, and the last was a normal mixed diet. The patients rotated through each of the diets. The subjects stayed in a hospital so they could be kept under constant observation to ensure strict dietary compliance.

Although the calorie consumption was exactly the same among each of the groups, the 90 percent fat diet (high-fat, low-carb) produced the greatest weight loss, followed closely by the 90 percent protein diet. Next came the mixed diet. Last of all was the very low-fat 90 percent carbohydrate diet.[7] In essence, the higher the carbohydrate content, the lower the weight loss and the higher the fat content, the greater the weight loss.

In a follow-up study, the researchers compared the weight loss of obese subjects on a high-carbohydrate diet with a high-fat diet, eating twice as many calories as in the previous study. Subjects on a high-carbohydrate 2,000-calorie diet failed to lose any weight. The same subjects on a high-fat diet not only lost weight at 2,000 calories, but lost weight even when calorie consumption increased to 2,600![8] A typical example of the subjects in this study was BJ. After eight days on the high-carbohydrate, 2,000-calorie diet, BJ didn't lose an ounce, but lost 9 pounds in 3 weeks on the 2,600-calorie, high-fat diet.

The researchers discovered that a high-fat diet stimulates the breakdown and burning of body fat, resulting in increased weight loss. Thus, adding fat into the diet stimulates the burning of body fat. Eating fat, it turns out, increases the body's utilization of stored fat, leading to weight loss. This is why eating fat caused greater weight loss than eating carbohydrate or protein.

This fat-burning effect can be so efficient that eating a calorie restricted, high-fat diet produces greater weight loss than eating nothing at all. Researchers at the US Naval Medical Research Institute compared two groups of overweight subjects; one group ate a high-fat diet, while the other group consumed no food at all. The subjects' weight loss over time was measured. The high-fat group consumed 1,000 calories a day, 90 percent of which came from fat. The remaining calories came from approximately 15 grams of protein and 10 grams of carbohydrate. The other group consumed no calories at all, only water. After ten days the fasting group lost 21 pounds on average, but most of that was from lean body tissue and water; only 7.5 pounds was from the loss of body fat. In comparison, the high-fat diet group lost on average 14.5 pounds, 14 of which was from body fat.[9] The group that ate 1,000 calories, mostly from fat, lost twice as much body fat as the group that ate nothing! Plus, they lost very little water and lean muscle. A reduced calorie diet with ample fat and limited carbohydrate will produce much greater weight loss than any low-fat diet, regardless of the number of calories consumed—even if this number is zero! Therefore, including an ample amount of fat in the diet is essential for greatest weight loss. This is a very important concept to remember for anyone trying to lose weight. You need to eat fat to lose fat.

Adding fat into a weight loss program will also make the diet much more satisfying and successful. The biggest stumbling block to successful dieting is the constant nagging hunger that accompanies it. It is hunger that drives dieters to cheat and eventually give up. Replacing some of the carbohydrate with fat produces a much greater feeling of satiety, with a higher degree of compliance and, consequently, success.

Dietary fat slows down the digestion of food, allowing the stomach to feel full longer and quenches the pangs of hunger. Fat stimulates the release of hormones that slow down the rate at which food leaves the stomach, allowing you to feel full longer. The small intestine also has fat receptors that act in much the same way. When you eat fatty foods you feel satisfied longer and don't sense a need to snack or to overeat at the next meal. This is a further reason why adding fat to your diet can help you lose weight!

In one study, for example, volunteers were given either a high-fat or a low-fat breakfast containing the same number of calories. Those who ate the high-fat breakfast felt full longer and delayed the time of their next meal, thus avoiding between meal snacks.[10]

Research has shown that when people get hungry soon after a meal, they tend to overeat at the next. Thus, a high-fat breakfast helps to prevent both between meal snacking and overeating. The end result is the consumption of fewer total calories. When used properly, fat can be an important aid in helping you lose weight and keeping it off.

Carbohydrate promotes fat storage and weight gain because it raises blood glucose, which stimulates a rise in insulin. Insulin promotes fat storage; the more insulin we have in our blood, the greater degree of fat storage occurs. Eating fat or protein does not cause a rise in blood glucose, and therefore, has a minor effect on insulin levels. If dietary carbohydrate consumption is kept low, eating fat does not contribute to weight gain because insulin levels are too low to promote fat storage. In fact, low insulin levels draw fat out of storage to be burned to produce energy. This is another yet reason why high-fat, low-carb diets are much more effective at managing weight than low-fat diets.

There have been a number of studies published that claim that high-fat diets promote weight gain and even insulin resistance and diabetes. However, these so-called high-fat diets are really high-carb diets with added fat. It is the carbohydrate in the diet that is causing the problem, but the blame is put on the fat. Carbohydrate triggers the release of insulin. Adding fat to a high-carb diet greatly increases the number of calories consumed. High insulin levels kick the body into fat storage mode so that these calories, whether from carbohydrate or fat, are packed away into storage. Therefore, when fat is added to a high-carb diet it can actually contribute to weight gain. To benefit from the weight-reducing effects of fat, the fat added into the diet must be accompanied by a decrease in carbohydrate intake. Doing this will allow total calorie intake to remain fairly consistent but produce beneficial results.

NUTRITIONAL SUPERFOOD

Fat is an important nutrient just as much as protein, vitamin C, or calcium, and is necessary to achieve and maintain good health. In the 1960s doctors began giving parenteral nutrition (nutrients delivered intravenously) to patients whose medical condition would not allow them to consume foods orally. Special nutritional formulas were designed to provide patients with all of the vitamins, minerals, electrolytes. amino acids, and carbohydrate to meet nutritional needs. Fatty acids were not included because it was believed the body could make all that was needed from the other nutrients. The formulas helped for a time, but without fat, patients eventually developed EFA deficiency; in infants and young children this was accompanied by growth impairment, developmental delays, dermatitis, and kidney and lung abnormalities. Adults also suffered from EFA deficiency. The addition of EFAs helped, but over time it was found that patients improved much faster when the formulas contained a mixture of saturated and unsaturated fatty acids.

In addition to serving as essential nutrients, fats serve another vital function. Fat fits the definition of a "functional food." These are special foods that provide health benefits above and beyond their basic nutritional content. Fat does much more than just supply a source of fatty acids. It makes other foods much more nutritious. Fat is necessary for the digestion and absorption of many essential nutrients in our diet. For example, it is through the fatty portion of foods that we get our fat-soluble nutrients, such as vitamins A, D, E, and K; CoQ_{10}; and the carotenoids (alpha-carotene, beta-carotene, lycopene, lutein, and others). These nutrients cannot be absorbed without adequate fat in the diet.

151

Dietary intake of foods rich in fat-soluble nutrients are associated with a reduced risk of a variety of common diseases including several types of cancer, cardiovascular disease, bladder disorders, kidney stones, fibrocystic breast disease, anemia, infections, macular degeneration, cataract, arthritis, and osteoporosis, to name a few. Many fat-soluble nutrients act as protective antioxidants, blocking the detrimental effects of destructive free radicals and AGEs and are involved in the regulation of cell growth, differentiation, and programmed cell death (apoptosis).

Fat improves the availability and absorption of almost all other nutrients as well. Fats slow down the movement of food through the stomach and digestive system. This allows more time for foods to bathe in stomach acids and digestive enzymes. As a consequence, more nutrients, including water-soluble vitamins such as the B vitamins, and minerals, which are normally tightly bound to other compounds, are released from our foods and absorbed into the body. While fats may not contain all these nutrients themselves, they make what nutrients that are in our foods more nutritious by increasing the absorption of their nutrient content.

Researchers at Purdue University fed volunteers salads that were topped with salad dressings containing three different quantities of fat—3, 8, or 20 grams. They also used three types of fat: butter, canola oil, and corn oil. Blood samples were taken from the subjects before and after eating to evaluate the amount of carotenoids absorbed into the bloodstream after the meal. The researchers discovered that the more fat the subjects consumed, the higher the carotenoid content in their blood, regardless of the type of fat consumed. Any source of fat improves nutrient absorption.[11]

How much of an effect does fat have on nutrient absorption? Apparently quite a lot. In a study conducted at Ohio State University, researchers looked at the absorption of four carotenoids (alpha-carotene, beta-carotene, lycopene, and lutein) in meals that had added fat. The researchers used avocado as the source of added fat.

Test subjects were given a meal of fat-free salsa and bread. On another day the same meal was given, but this time avocado was added to the salsa, boosting the fat content of the meal to about 37 percent of calories. Blood levels of the test subjects showed that beta-carotene increased 2.6 times and lycopene 4.4 times, demonstrating that adding a little fat to the meal can more than double, triple, or quadruple nutrient absorption.

The researchers performed a second test in which the subjects ate salads with varying amounts of fat. The first salad included romaine lettuce, baby spinach, shredded carrots, and a non-fat dressing, resulting in a fat content of about 2 percent. The fat content was increased with three additional salads consumed on different days, containing either 75 grams of avocado, 150 grams of avocado, or 24 grams of avocado oil (a little under 5 teaspoons). As the fat content of the salad increased, so did the absorption of the carotenoids, with the greatest increase occurring with the addition of the avocado oil. The highest fat salad increased blood levels of lutein 6.7 times, alpha-carotene 8.9 times, and beta-carotene an impressive 17.4 times! According to this study, adding fat to salad vegetables increases the amount of nutrition you get from them by as much as 1,740 percent! Now, that is what I call a functional superfood![12]

The researchers were surprised not only by how adding fat improved nutrient absorption, but also by how little is absorbed in the absence of fat. If you want to get all the nutrients you can from a tomato, green beans, spinach, or any vegetable or low-fat food, you need to add some fat. Eating vegetables without added fat is in effect the same as eating a nutritionally poor meal. Adding a good source of fat in the diet is important to gaining the most nutrition from your foods.

Fat is what can make other superfoods like kale, broccoli, spinach, and seaweed so powerful. Most superfoods are naturally low in fat, and eating them without a source of added fat greatly diminishes the availability of the nutrients they contain, making them no better than any ordinary food. Without fat, these so-called superfoods are no longer very super. It is the added fat that allows them to reach their superfood potential.

Many of the fat-soluble vitamins function as antioxidants that protect us from free-radical damage. Free-radical chemical reactions within our bodies cause the destruction of cells and their DNA. Free radicals are continually being formed inside our bodies and are associated with most every known acute and degenerative disease. Many researchers believe that free-radical reactions are a primary cause of aging. The more free-radical damage your body sustains, the faster you age. By reducing the amount of fat in your diet, you limit the amount of protective antioxidant nutrients available to protect you from destructive free-radical reactions. Low-fat diets speed the process of degeneration and aging. This may be one of the reasons why those people who stay on very low-fat diets for any length of time often look pale, sickly, and much older than they really are.

Carotenoids are fat-soluble nutrients found in fruits and vegetables. The best known is beta-carotene. All of the carotenoids are known for their antioxidant capability. Many studies have shown them and other fat-soluble antioxidants, such as vitamins A and E, to provide protection from degenerative conditions and to support immune system function.

Vegetables such as broccoli and carrots have beta-carotene, but if you don't eat any oil with them, you won't get the full benefit of the fat-soluble vitamins they contain. If you eat a salad with low-fat dressing or you omit other sources of fat, like avocado or nuts, you lose most of the vitamins present in the vegetables.

Another important nutrient that needs fat for proper absorption is calcium. You can drink loads of nonfat milk and low-fat cheese and shovel down calcium supplements but still develop osteoporosis. Why? Because calcium needs fat in order to be absorbed. If you drink nonfat milk for the calcium, you are wasting your money. You need whole milk and full-fat cheese and other full-fat foods in order to absorb the calcium. Many vegetables are also good sources of calcium. But to take advantage of that calcium, you need to eat them with butter and cream or other foods that contain fat.

Instead of harming the heart, fat feeds the heart and supports healthy heart function. The heart's preferred source of energy is not glucose, but fat, particularly saturated fat. Fats are good for your heart and circulatory system. This was shown in a study conducted by nutritionist Mary Flynn, PhD. Twenty subjects were given a diet with 37 percent of the calories from fat, and she measured their cholesterol and triglyceride levels. She then gave the same group a diet with less fat—25 percent of calories, but kept the total number of calories exactly the same by increasing carbohydrates. She found that the low-fat diet lowered levels of good HDL cholesterol (a move considered bad for the heart and circulatory system), raised triglyceride levels (also considered bad), and basically left the levels of bad LDL cholesterol unchanged (neither good nor bad).[13] The overall effect was bad for the heart. You combine this with the fact that fat-soluble vitamins, such as vitamin E and beta-carotene, which help protect against heart disease, are reduced in a low-fat diet, and you see that low-fat diets may actually promote heart disease—just the opposite from what we are led to believe.

One of the recognized risk factors for heart disease is elevated homocysteine levels. Homocysteine levels rise when there is a deficiency of vitamins B_6, B_{12}, or folic acid. Consuming an adequate amount of fat with your foods will improve the absorption of these three B vitamins, helping protect against elevated homocysteine levels, and consequently, heart disease.

Vitamin A is a fat-soluble nutrient that is most well-known for its association with eye health. The vitamin is necessary for the proper function of the lens, cornea, and retina. A deficiency can lead to a form of retinopathy that causes night blindness. Left untreated, it can lead to permanent vision loss. Vitamin A deficiency is the number-one cause of childhood blindness in the world. One of the functions of vitamin A is that of an antioxidant, and provides protection to the lens against free-radical damage that can lead to cataracts—the primary cause of vision loss in adults worldwide. Vitamin A deficiency can also cause growth and mental retardation, lower immune function, and dry out mucous membranes.

We get vitamin A from fats in *animal* products. Good sources include beef liver, cod liver oil, oysters, whole milk, cream, cheese, butter, eggs, and fatty meat. You may have heard claims that carrots are good for the eyes because they contain vitamin A. Technically, this is not true, as only animal products contain vitamin A; however, plants do contain carotenoids, many of which can be converted by our bodies into vitamin A. In fact, the vitamin A we get from animals was once the carotenoids found in the grass, leaves, and other plants they ate. When these plants were eaten by an animal, some of the carotenoids were converted into vitamin A. Vitamin A tends to collect in fatty tissues.

Carotenoids are plant pigments that give red, yellow, orange, and green fruits and vegetables much of their color. The red color in tomatoes comes from carotenoids, as well as the orange color in carrots. A carotenoid that can be converted into vitamin A is called provitamin A or vitamin A precursor. The efficiency in which carotenoids are transformed into vitamin A is low, so a much higher amount of carotenoids must be consumed to equal the amount of vitamin A you get from animal sources. Beta-carotene is the carotenoid that has the highest conversion rate. It takes about 12 times as much beta-carotene, by weight, to equal the amount of vitamin A from animal sources and about 24 times as much of the other provitamin A carotenoids (alpha-carotene, gamma-carotene, and beta-cryptoxanthin) to do the same.

Foods that are good sources of carotenoids are fruits and vegetables with rich red, orange, yellow, and green colors such as leafy green vegetables (spinach, chard, turnip greens, bok choy, etc.), carrots, sweet potatoes, butternut squash, mangos, tomatoes, parsley, apricots, broccoli, red cabbage, and asparagus.

Unfortunately, eating foods rich in carotenoids is not necessarily enough to ward off vitamin A deficiency. Vitamin A is a fat-soluble nutrient. In order to effectively convert beta-carotene or any other provitamin A carotenoid into vitamin A, an adequate amount of fat must also be consumed at the same time. Eating beta-carotene with fat can improve the conversion rate sixfold. In other words, when consumed with an adequate amount of fat you only need twice as much beta-carotene, rather than 12 times as much, to equal the amount of vitamin A you get in animal foods. Most vegetables and fruits do not contain enough fat for efficient conversion, so a person can eat large amounts of carotenoid-rich vegetables and fruits, yet still suffer from a vitamin A deficiency. For example, in Asia, many children eat diets containing what should be adequate amounts of provitamin A carotenoids, but due to poverty, they don't combine it with enough good sources of fat, such as milk, eggs, animal fat, nuts, coconut, or vegetable oils (palm, olive, and coconut). Consequently, they often suffer from vitamin A deficiency.

Likewise, we can eat a bowl full of carotenoid-rich fruits and vegetables, but without added fat, not enough vitamin A will be made from it to meet our needs.

One of the major problems with low-fat foods and low-fat diets is that they can create a nutrient deficiency. In order for your body to assimilate the nutrients in your foods, you need to eat them with a source of fat. If you don't eat enough fat, these nutrients will pass right though the digestive tract doing you little good. For this reason, low-fat diets are dangerous. Eating a low-fat diet for any length of time can lead to nutritional deficiencies that can greatly increase your risk for disease and premature aging.

Fat is the only superfood that can transform carotenoids into vitamin A and improve the absorption of all of the other nutrients in our foods. When you add fats to your meals, your foods become far more nutritious; it is like adding a natural, high-potency, full-spectrum, vitamin, mineral, and antioxidant supplement to your diet.

PROTECTION FROM INFECTION

We live in a sea of microorganisms; they are in the air we breathe, the food we eat, the water we drink, and even live on our bodies. Some of these microbes are relatively harmless and can even be beneficial, while others can cause sickness and death. For the most part, our immune system protects us from infection by the more malevolent varieties.

When an infant is born, it comes from the relatively sterile environment of the womb into a world that is teeming with potentially harmful germs. At this stage of life the immune system is not fully developed and the infant is highly vulnerable to infection. Fortunately, infants are not born defenseless; mother's milk contains several substances that protect infants from infections during this critical time. Some protection comes from the mother's antibodies in her milk, but perhaps the greatest protection comes from its fat content.

Mother's milk is rich in fats, mostly saturated and monounsaturated fats, with some polyunsaturated fat to supply the infant's EFA needs. These fats serve multiple functions; they provide nourishment, help to establish a healthy gut microbiome, and ward off infection and disease.

Long chain fatty acids (LCFAs) from our foods modulate intestinal immune function, which is independent of the systemic immune system. The absorption of LCFAs stimulates the influx of lymphocytes, a type of white blood cell, through the intestinal wall. This process helps defend against potentially harmful microorganisms that may have found entry into the gastrointestinal tract from the meal.[14] Germs can be carried into the body by any type of food—milk, vegetables, fruits, grains, and so forth. Including some fat with meals helps protect against infection. Mother's milk naturally supplies the fat necessary to do this.

In addition, many fatty acids, especially those in breast milk, possess potent antimicrobial properties capable of killing troublesome bacteria, viruses, fungi, and parasites. These fatty acids are powerful enough to kill intestinal troublemakers like E. coli, H. pylori, and *Candida albicans*, yet are completely harmless to human cells. Unlike antibiotics that kill all bacteria, fatty acids are more selective, they can kill the major troublemakers yet leave the good bacteria alone. In this way, potential troublemakers are suppressed while the good microbes are allowed to thrive and firmly establish themselves in the infant's digestive tract, producing a healthy gut microbiome.

As you recall from Chapter 7, the fats we eat are composed of triglycerides. Triglycerides consist of three fatty acids joined together by a glycerol molecule. When fats are consumed and digested, the triglycerides are gradually broken down into diglycerides (two fatty acids joined by a glycerol), monoglycerides (one fatty acid attached to a glycerol), and individual fatty acids. It is the monoglycerides and fatty acids that have the antimicrobial properties. Triglycerides and diglycerides have none.

Some fatty acids are more effective at killing certain types of microorganisms than others. Some kill bacteria like E. coli, others kill streptococcus and staphylococcus, and still others yeasts and viruses. For example, capric acid, a 10 chain saturated fatty acid, is more effective at killing certain bacteria than caprylic acid, an 8 chain saturated fatty acid; however, caprylic acid is more effective at killing certain fungi than capric acid. Natural fats contain a mixture of several different types of fatty acids, so they are effective against a wide variety of pathogens.

The antimicrobial effect varies greatly among the different fatty acids. Some are very potent while others are rather weak (see table on the following page). Medium chain fatty acids display the greatest antimicrobial activity, with lauric acid and its monoglyceride—monolaurin—having the strongest overall effect. Medium chain triglycerides are important components of mother's milk. MCFAs also stimulate the production of white blood cells, boosting immune function. These and other fatty acids are essential in establishing the infant's gut microbiome and provide protection from systemic infections.

Adults also benefit in a similar manner from the antimicrobial properties of fatty acids through the consumption of fats and oils. After weaning, we no longer enjoy the benefits of mother's milk and the MCTs it contains, but we can get MCTs through the consumption of dairy, as all mammal milks contain these protective fats. Other than dairy, there are very few good

Minimal Inhibitory Concentration of Fatty Acids

Fatty acid	Pneumococci	Streptococcus Group A	Streptococcus betahemolytic non-A	Candida albicans	S. aureus
Caproic	NI	NI	NI	NI	NI
Caprylic	NI	NI	NI	NI	NI
Capric	1.45	1.45	2.9	2.9	2.9
Lauric	0.062	0.124	0.249	0.249	0.249
Myristic	0.218	0.547	2.18	4.37	4.37
Myristoleic	0.110	0.110	0.110	0.552	0.441
Palmitic	0.48	3.9	3.0	NI	NI
Palmitoleic	0.024	0.098	0.049	0.491	0.983
Stearic	NI	NI	NI	NI	NI
Oleic	NI	NI	NI	NI	NI
Elaidic	NI	NI	NI	NI	NI
Linoleic	0.044	0.089	0.089	0.455	NI
Linolenic	0.179	0.35	0.35	NI	1.79
Arachidonic	NI	NI	NI	NI	NI

The antimicrobial potency of fatty acids varies by concentration. The lower the concentration needed to inhibit the growth of the microbe, the stronger the effect. In the table above, the smaller the number, the stronger the antimicrobial effect. The results in the table are given in mM. NI=not inhibitory at the concentrations tested (1.0 mg/ml or 3 to 6.0 mM). Source: Kabara, J. J. (ed). The Pharmacological Effect of Lipids. The American Oil Chemists' Society: Champaign, Illinois, 1978.

dietary sources for MCTs. The best natural sources are coconut and palm kernel oils. Coconut oil is by far the richest natural source, with even more than that found in mother's milk. Coconut oil is composed of 63 percent MCFAs, with lauric acid comprising almost 50 percent. Palm kernel oil contains 53 percent MCFAs, with lauric acid making up about 45 percent. In comparison, butter, which is the third richest source, contains only 8 percent MCFAs. Most of the other fatty acids possess varying degrees of antimicrobial fighting power and when consumed together, work synergistically to help protect us from infection.

Germs are everywhere. No matter how hard you try to scrub your dishes, clean your hands, and wash your food, germs are always present. Acids in our stomach kill most germs, but some manage to slip by to disrupt the gut microbiome or cause illness. The fats in our foods act as a secondary means of protection. In the digestive tract they destroy disease-causing organisms on contact. Fatty acids in the bloodstream help fight off systemic infections.

Unlike antibiotics, which kill only bacteria, fatty acids are effective against bacteria as well as viruses, fungi, and some parasites. For generations mothers have given their families homemade chicken soup to fight off the cold or flu (viral infections). As it turns out, a handful of scientific studies show that chicken soup really could have medicinal value.[15-17] Although these studies do not identify the exact ingredient or ingredients in the soups that make them effective, it might possibly be the fat. Homemade chicken soup is generally a rich source of fat.

So, when you eat a meal containing fat, you are eating food that will protect you from many forms of food poisoning and infectious disease. If, on the other hand, you avoid fat and eat low-fat foods, you are making it easier for germs to survive in your digestive tract and cause trouble. A truly healthy diet will always include ample amounts of fat.

Having a healthy gut microbiome promotes good digestive health. An imbalance in the microbiota can lead to chronic inflammation and a variety of gastrointestinal problems such as leaky gut syndrome, irritable bowel syndrome (IBS), Crohn's disease, and ulcerative colitis, to name a few. Dietary fats help keep the microbiome in balance and avoid these types of conditions.

Researchers at Case Western Reserve University School of Medicine have shown a high-fat diet may lead to specific changes in gut bacteria that could fight harmful inflammation and ease conditions such as Crohn's disease. Crohn's, a type of inflammatory bowel disease, causes debilitating intestinal swelling, cramping, and diarrhea.

In the study, a diet of "good" fats, which included coconut oil and cocoa butter, drastically reduced certain types of bacteria in mice with Crohn's-like disease. Both these fats have a high amount of saturated fatty acids, and coconut oil is predominantly medium chain fatty acids. Mice fed beneficial fatty diets had up to 30 percent fewer kinds of gut bacteria as those fed a normal diet, collectively resulting in a very different gut microbial composition. Some of the species changes showed up in feces, while others were different in the cecum, a portion of the intestine commonly inflamed in Crohn's disease. Mice fed even low concentrations of coconut oil or cocoa butter also had less severe small intestine inflammation.

"The finding is remarkable because it means that a Crohn's patient could also have a beneficial effect on their gut bacteria and inflammation by only switching the type of fat in their diet," said Alexander Rodriguez-Palacios,

PhD, one of the coauthors of the study. "Patients would only need to replace a 'bad' fat with a 'good' fat, and eat normal amounts."

The study is one of the first to identify specific changes in gut bacteria associated with Crohn's disease. It is also the first to show how high-fat diets can alter gut bacteria to combat inflammation. Results from the study could help doctors identify bacteria to use in probiotics to treat patients suffering from inflammatory bowel syndromes.[18]

Dietary fats protect us from systemic infections as well. Saturated fats, and particularly lauric acid, increase the production of HDL cholesterol.[19-20] This is important because HDL has been shown to help protect against cardiovascular disease, reduce inflammation, and aid the immune system in fighting infections. HDL plays an important role in our defense by absorbing endotoxins produced by bacteria and transporting them to the liver where they are neutralized and excreted from the body.[21-22] Much of the harm caused by bacterial infections comes from the deleterious effects of the endotoxins they produce. HDL mops up these toxins and clears them from the body. Both animal and human studies have shown that higher HDL levels increase resistance to and reduce the risk of death from bacterial infections.[23-24] HDL is not only protective against bacteria but has also been shown to inhibit the ability of certain viruses to penetrate our cells and to play an important role in defending against parasitic infections. Eating saturated fat or a low-carb diet have both been shown to be the most effective ways to increase HDL levels.

IMMUNE FUNCTION

The antimicrobial properties of dietary fats help train our immune system during infancy and keep it in good working order throughout life.

When we eat a meal, protein is broken down into amino acids and fat is broken down into fatty acids, making them small enough to penetrate the intestinal wall. Inside the intestinal wall, fatty acids and amino acids are combined into little bundles of fat and protein called *chylomicrons*. These chylomicrons travel from the lymphatic system to the bloodstream, where they circulate throughout the body delivering fat and protein to wherever they are needed.

As triglycerides are broken down in the gastrointestinal tract, fatty acids are released. Certain saturated and unsaturated fatty acids kill potentially troublesome bacteria. Many of the bacteria that are destroyed have an outer cell membrane composed of lipopolysaccharides (LPS). Some LPS fragments from the destroyed bacteria are small enough to pass through the epithelial lining and into the intestinal wall. Here the fragments are picked up with fatty acids, amino acids, and other substances and packaged into chylomicrons and eventually carried into circulation.[25]

In the bloodstream, LPS is recognized as a foreign invader—a bacterium—and stimulates an immune response. Because of this process, some researchers have suggested that eating high-fat diets promotes systemic inflammation leading to the development of obesity, diabetes, heart disease, and other disorders accompanied by chronic inflammation. They claim that dietary fat, particularly saturated fat, is inflammatory, and therefore causes chronic inflammatory related disease. In their zeal to find reasons to condemn dietary fat, the obvious is overlooked.

Fat has always been an important part of the human diet. Some populations, such as the Inuit, native Siberians, the Maasai of Africa, and many others subsisted and thrived on very high-fat diets. Over the past century thousands of people have adopted a very high-fat, ketogenic diet, some for extended periods lasting many years, and have not experienced obesity, diabetes, or heart disease. In fact, just the opposite happens; those on ketogenic diets generally lose excess weight, develop better blood sugar control, and reduce their risk of heart disease. The high-fat diet didn't harm them, but made them healthier.

Fats are essential in establishing a healthy gut microbiome in newborn infants and in maintaining a healthy microbial population throughout life. The absorption of LPS is a normal and universal process that occurs in both humans and animals.[26] It is not a defect in biology or some freakish abnormality caused by eating fat. In animals, the process is the same. Carnivores and some omnivores, for example, eat a lot of meat and fat but do not become obese or develop diabetes or heart disease. However, dogs and cats fed pet foods high in processed grains, soy, and other carbohydrates with only moderate fat, often do develop these human diseases. Obviously, meat and fat·do not cause these problems in animals or in humans.

In the body, when a white blood cell senses the presence of LPS, it interprets it as an invasion by potentially harmful bacteria and initiates an immune reaction by activating an inflammatory response and stimulating the production of more white blood cells to defend the body. This is the body's normal reaction to a potential threat. Contrary to popular belief, inflammation isn't something that is bad or evil, it is the normal process in which the body mounts a defense and fights off infection. In most cases, it is a good thing, as it is protecting the body. Only when inflammation becomes chronic and never shuts down does it become a problem. This only happens when there is a stimulus that constantly triggers inflammation, such as chronic infection or tissue irritation. The slight inflammatory reaction from LPS after eating fat is usually only temporary and not a chronic condition even

161

when fat is consumed at every meal. Interestingly, people who have been on very high-fat diets (60-80 percent of total calories consumed) for a while generally have optimal C-reactive protein (CRP) levels. CRP is a marker for systemic inflammation. Those people who are diabetic, overweight, or at high risk for heart disease, have distinctively elevated CPR levels, indicating chronic inflammation.

While the consumption of some types of fatty acids do raise blood levels of LPS, markers for inflammation remain unchanged, indicating that high-fat meals do not trigger systemic inflammation, although there may be an increase in white blood cell production.[27] LPS can stimulate an inflammatory response, especially when it is associated with living bacteria, but apparently when the source of the LPS follows a fatty meal there is little or no accompanying inflammatory response.

These LPS fragments trigger a mild immune response, which includes the increased production of white blood cells. White blood cells are the workhorse of our immune system and an increase in their numbers enhances immune function. More immune cells on the job means more cells are at work, seeking out and eliminating all potentially harmful troublemakers, not just bacteria, but viruses, yeasts, parasites, toxins, cancerous cells, and LPS fragments.

Instead of being a defect caused by a high-fat diet, the absorption of gut-derived LPS fragments is a normal and even necessary process of biology. LPS makes up the outer cell membrane of many pathogenic bacteria and is not the whole living organism. LPS is often used in medical research as a means to stimulate an immune response without the threat of causing an actual infection. Unlike living bacteria, it can't multiply and grow. It is defenseless against the immune system.

For this reason, LPS provides a valuable tool to condition and train the immune system without danger. This is especially important in infants, whose immune systems are still developing and learning how to recognize harmful substances. Nursing infants eat a very high-fat diet. About 56 percent of the calorie content in human breast milk comes from fat, half of which is saturated fat. Many of these fats have the ability to kill potentially harmful bacteria in the gut. LPS fragments from the dead bacteria are then absorbed into the bloodstream and initiate a mild immune response. This way the infant's immune system is trained to recognize harmful microorganisms. The slight increase in white blood cells boosts immune efficiency and the clearance of microbes and toxins from the bloodstream. This process continues in adults, keeping the immune system sharp and ready to leap into action whenever living invaders enter the bloodstream.[28]

LPS in large numbers, due to an active infection, can make you sick, but the tiny amount that enters the bloodstream from the digestive tract is too small to cause any noticeable symptoms or any harm. The release of LPS into the body from the gut is a normal, natural, harmless process. It couldn't be otherwise, as this process occurs in all infants. The fats in mother's milk are there to nourish and protect the infant, not to cause its early demise. Dietary fat serves a very important role in training and maintaining proper immune function.

DIGESTIVE HEALTH

We have already seen how dietary fats can help regulate the types of microbiota that live in the gastrointestinal tract. Keeping the microbes that inhabit the intestines in balance is very important to good digestive health. Another important aspect to consider is the nutritional health of your intestines. You can have lots of good bacteria living in the digestive tract, but if the intestines themselves are malnourished and sickly, you will not absorb nutrients effectively and may develop inflammatory bowel disease or other digestive problems.

The digestion and absorption process is critically dependent on energy; the digestive system (intestines, pancreas, spleen, and stomach) makes up less than 6 percent of the body's weight but consumes up to 35 percent of the body's energy. The cells in the intestines never sleep, never go on vacation, never take a break; they are continually active and need a continual supply of energy to function properly and remain healthy. Where do your intestines get their energy? Much of it comes from fat. Believe it or not, your intestines thrive on fat.

The most important source of fat for your intestines comes from short chain fatty acids (SCFAs).[29] While a small amount of SCFAs are found in the diet, primarily in dairy fat, the most important source comes from bacteria within the gastrointestinal tract. Certain gut bacteria breakdown the dietary fiber in our foods into SCFAs. The otherwise indigestible fiber contained in the vegetables, fruits, grains, and seeds is transformed into SCFAs. We do not have the capability to break down this fiber because we lack the enzymes needed. However, gut bacteria can break them down, forming the SCFAs butyrate (C4), propionate (C3), and acetate (C2). SCFAs are the primary food or fuel used by the epithelial cells lining the lower portion of your intestinal tract. Unlike glucose, which requires the aid of insulin to enter the cells and be converted into energy, SCFAs easily diffuse through the intestinal cell membrane without the need of insulin, providing a quick and easy source of fuel. SCFAs provide 60 to 70 percent of the energy consumed by the epithelial cells in the colon.

At first, you might think it odd that dietary fiber can be so easily converted into fat. However, it is not unusual at all considering that fiber is a carbohydrate and the liver converts carbohydrate into fat all the time.

SCFAs are important to the health of your intestines and the integrity of the intestinal wall. Without them, the epithelial lining of the digestive tract would begin to degenerate; the cells would literally starve to death. This would cause chronic inflammation and tissue breakdown, which could lead to leaky gut syndrome, lesions or ulcers, ulcerative colitis, Crohn's disease, and other digestive disorders. Nutrient absorption could also be dramatically affected, leading to malnutrition. It is quite possible that many people suffering from inflammatory bowel disease are really suffering from a malnourished digestive tract.

Our modern diet is woefully deficient in dietary fiber. Sugar contains no fiber. Refined grains are almost completely devoid of it. The small amount of fiber in the diet may be enough to keep the intestinal cells from total starvation, but not healthy. A diet lacking an adequate amount of high-fiber foods can lead to various forms of digestive stress as well as malnutrition.

SCFAs do much more than just provide food for intestinal epithelial cells. Recent research reveals that they play a key role in the prevention and treatment of metabolic syndrome, insulin resistance and diabetes, bowel disorders, and colon cancer.[30-33] SCFAs lower the colonic pH (i.e., raise the acidity level in the colon), which provides a suitable environment for helpful microbiota, protects the lining from forming colonic polyps, and increases absorption of dietary minerals. They stimulate the production of T-helper cells, leukocytes, and antibodies, which play crucial roles in immune protection. They have anti-inflammatory effects and can help ease inflammation in the digestive tract caused by microbiota dysbiosis, ulcers, injuries, and such. In clinical studies SCFAs have been used therapeutically for the successful treatment of ulcerative colitis, Crohn's disease, and antibiotic-associated diarrhea.[34-36]

SCFAs aren't the only types of fat intestinal cells consume. They also love MCFAs—the same ones found in coconut oil, mother's milk, and dairy products. MCFAs in human breast milk serve many purposes. They provide a source of nutrition for the infant, feed intestinal epithelial cells, kill potentially harmful microbiota, calm inflammation, and do basically everything else associated with SCFAs noted earlier. This may be why dietary MCFAs from coconut oil have such a positive effect on many bowel disorders.

MCFAs may be even more beneficial than SCFAs in many aspects of digestive health. SCFAs have some mild antimicrobial effects, but MCFAs are much more potent and can kill many potentially troublesome microorganisms and help maintain a healthy intestinal ecology. Just like SCFAs, MCFAs also easily diffuse through the epithelial cell membrane, without the need of insulin. Studies have shown that MCFAs are absorbed even better than SCFAs.[37] The addition of coconut oil to the diet can provide a nutritional boost to colon health. Combined with its antimicrobial and anti-inflammatory properties, this may be one of the reasons coconut oil and other coconut products have been reported to have such a positive effect on gastrointestinal health. Studies support this observation. For instance, a number of studies have experimentally induced colitis in animals using toxic chemicals administered by an enema. Feeding the animals a diet containing MCFAs has shown to significantly reduce inflammation and damage caused by these toxins.[38-39] MCFAs can help with colitis caused by other conditions as well. In the study on inflammatory bowel disease, instead of using toxic chemicals to induce injury, researchers can use genetically bred mice that spontaneously develop chronic intestinal inflammation and deep ulcers that resemble Crohn's disease in humans. When MCFAs are added to the animal's diet, there is a marked decrease in the incidence of colitis and a reduction in inflammatory markers.[40] Studies on humans with Crohn's disease have shown the addition of MCTs in hospital feeding formulas can induce clinical remission.[41-42]

Coconut and palm kernel oils consist of about 63 and 53 percent MCFAs, respectively. Milk fat contains both SCFAs and MCFAs. Butter is composed of 4 percent SCFAs, principally butyrate, and 8 percent MCFAs. The remaining 88 percent of the fatty acids are LCFAs. The fats in most meats and plant foods are 100 percent LCFAs. These long chain fats can also provide fuel for the intestinal cells, but not like MCFAs or SCFAs do. Like glucose, the longer chain fatty acids require insulin to pass through a cell membrane and serve as fuel.

When you eat fats containing long chain triglycerides, they are slowly broken down into individual fatty acids in the small intestine. When a triglyceride is fully digested, it produces one glycerol molecule and three fatty acids. The glycerol is an organic alcohol. If the fatty acids are short chain or medium chain, they can be used to feed the intestinal cells. The long chain fatty acids cannot; they are absorbed into the intestinal lining and eventually released into the bloodstream. However, glycerol, like short and medium chain fatty acids, can pass through the intestinal cell membrane easily and be converted into energy without the aid of insulin.[43] In addition, some bacteria consume glycerol and produce butyric acid. As triglycerides travel down the digestive tract, glycerol is being released, providing an additional source of food for the gut wall and the resident bacteria. For this reason, a high-fat diet can be very nourishing for the digestive tract and even provide some of the nourishment the epithelium needs in the absence of dietary fiber. While the intestines thrive on fat, not all fats are alike. Doctors often recommend a low-fat diet for patients with inflammatory bowel disorders. One of the reasons for this is that too much polyunsaturated fats, rich in linoleic acid, can make these conditions worse. Linoleic acid is pro-inflammatory and can aggravate inflammatory conditions.[44] Linoleic acid is the primary fatty acid in most polyunsaturated vegetables oils, such as corn and soybean oils, two of the most widely used oils in the food industry. For this reason, saturated and monounsaturated fats are preferred for digestive health.

The health of your gastrointestinal tract not only affects digestive function but also other aspects of your health and life. Research shows that the condition of the digestive system has a direct influence on mental health and mood, hormones, bone density, joint health, glucose metabolism, body weight, blood sugar levels, kidney function, and so much more.[45-52] Eating enough of the right types of fat and good sources of fiber can have a very pronounced effect on digestive function and your overall health.

IMPROVED PHYSICAL AND MENTAL PERFORMANCE

The foods we eat can have a marked effect on our mental health. Our nervous system contains a very high percentage of fat; our brains are 60 percent fat. It is only reasonable to assume that the amount of fat in our diet can affect our mental health. If so, then the diets of people whose jobs affect the lives and safety of others must be of the best quality to assure top mental performance. This was the focus of a study commissioned by the U.S. military.

The study tracked 45 student pilots to assess how different foods affected the pilots' mental performance. Every three weeks, each pilot spent one week on one of four different diets: high-fat, high-carbohydrate, high-protein, and a control diet. The diets were given to each pilot in random order and the menus were similar so the type of diet wouldn't be obvious to the participants.[53]

The study used a flight simulator that required students to navigate and descend in cloudy weather when the runway wasn't visible and using only the plane's computers. They also took tests that required memorizing and repeating numbers and comparing shapes. Although the pilots did not know the difference in the foods, they did notice the difference in their own performance. "I could tell the difference on how well I was doing on the different diets," said Jeremy Ternes, one of the student pilots. "There were times I thought, Wow, I was a lot more on today as compared to last week."

Based on the pilots' test scores, the researchers found that those who ate the fattiest foods, such as butter and gravy, had the quickest response times in mental tests and made the fewest mistakes when flying in challenging conditions. The pilots' mental performance was significantly better with the high-fat diet over the other diets. This was an important finding because it may help decrease the number of aviation accidents due to pilot error, which is especially important for the combat fighter.

It is also important for the non-pilot as well. It means that getting adequate fat into the diet is important for proper mental function. Students could do better in school and adults would perform better at their jobs and perhaps there would also be fewer automobile accidents.

Not only is the mind sharper and reflexes quicker, but physical endurance and athletic performance can improve with a high-fat diet in comparison with a lower-fat diet. This was demonstrated by Peter J. Horvath, PhD, associate professor in the Department of Physical Therapy, Exercise and Nutrition Sciences at the University of Buffalo, New York. His early research found that both male and female competitive runners showed improved athletic performance on higher-fat diets. This led him to investigate how dietary fat can affect women athletes.

His study involved nine female collegiate soccer players who ate three diets in a randomized crossover design: (1) their normal diet, which served as the control; (2) their normal diet plus 415 calories of oil-roasted peanuts per day; and (3) their normal diet plus 415 calories from a carbohydrate-rich energy bar. The high-fat diet supplied 35 percent of calories as fat, the high-carb diet 24 percent as fat, and the normal diet 27 percent. The women consumed each diet for seven days.

Endurance testing was designed to mimic soccer play, using constant speed running and running at different rates on a treadmill, plus forward running with a side-step maneuver performed on a force plate. The athletes were tested until exhaustion on the seventh day of each diet. Treadmill speed increased progressively, which meant the longer the athletes performed, the harder they had to work.

The results showed that the soccer players were able to perform longer at a higher intensity on the highest-fat diet, with no lessening of muscle performance, as measured by the force plate. As fat calories decreased, so did performance. The lowest-fat diet with the high-carb energy bar, despite the added carb calories, produced the worst results.

"When women consumed the high-fat diet, they performed longer at the highest intensity," Horvath said. Distances were 11.2 km on the high-fat diet, 10 km on the normal diet, and 9.7 km on the high-carbohydrate diet.

"The women went 1.2 to 1.5 kilometers farther before reaching exhaustion while doing very-high-speed intermittent exercise when on the high-fat diet, compared to the lower-fat diets," said Horvath. "That is really a striking difference."

"These results support our thesis that supplementing the diets of female athletes with peanuts or other fat sources can help build up their energy reserves and improve performance," Horvath said. "A low-fat diet may result in a poorer performance for women in a long, intermittently intense sport like soccer."[54]

Low-fat diets can be detrimental for both mental and physical performance. Fat is essential for healthy nerve function. Good nerve health is important for quick reflexes in sports, piloting a jet fighter, or even just driving your car.

Nerve cells have a main body with many short arms called *dendrites* and one very long arm called the *axon*. Messages are passed from cell to cell through the axon on one nerve cell to the dendrites of another. Whether by conscious thought or from a subconscious reflex, nerve impulses are sent to and from the brain this way. Many of the nerves in both our central and peripheral nervous systems have a specialized fat- and cholesterol-rich coating covering the axon, called a *myelin sheath*. This fatty coating acts as an insulator, which greatly increases the speed at which nerve impulses travel from cell to cell. Fat is essential for making the myelin sheath and a dietary deficiency could affect nerve function, which in turn could affect mental function and reaction time. For this reason, eating enough fat is important for sharp physical performance.

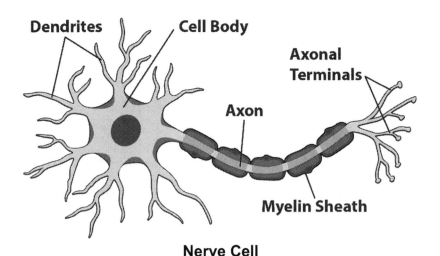

Nerve Cell

Another reason fat is advantageous in sports is that it supplies an additional source of energy to glucose. For many years coaches and trainers have instructed athletes to load up on carbohydrates to achieve peak physical performance. Carbohydrate is needed to fill their glycogen stores so they will have the energy to sustain them for the duration of their training and competition. Glucose is stored in the muscles in the form of glycogen and allows the muscles to access glucose quickly. The concept that a diet high in carbohydrate is necessary for optimizing exercise performance was recognized in the late 1960s when it was discovered that muscle glycogen depletion was associated with fatigue, and that a high-carbohydrate diet maintained muscle glycogen and performance. Endurance athletes talk about "hitting the wall" during competition. This term refers to the point at which glycogen stores are completely depleted and the muscles have no glucose to burn. Continued physical exertion becomes extremely arduous. Athletes had to resort to carbohydrate loading before an event and consume additional sources of carbohydrate during and afterward to avoid total glycogen depletion.

Humans possess a robust capacity to adapt to low-carbohydrate availability and switch to using fat as fuel. When glycogen levels significantly decrease, fatty acids are utilized to supply the majority of energy needed by the muscles.

Fat has a greater capacity to store energy than glucose; and the fat we carry on our bodies is far more plentiful than the glycogen stored in our muscles and liver. For example, a 175-pound (80 kg) man with 15 percent body fat, stores about 350 grams of glycogen in his skeletal muscles, providing 1,200 calories of energy. During endurance races these calories are eventually used up, and consuming carbohydrate during the event can replenish some of these calories and keep him going. In comparison, the fat stored on the same size man can provide up to 92,000 calories of energy, greatly enhancing his capacity for endurance, and slow the depletion of his glycogen stores. For this reason, many endurance athletes have switched from a high-carbohydrate to a low-carbohydrate, high-fat diet with great success.

When the diet is high is carbohydrate, the body tends to rely almost exclusively on glucose for fuel, severely limiting access to the abundant supply of energy from available fat.[55] For this reason, most people cannot switch immediately from a high-carb to a low-carb, high-fat diet and maintain the same level of performance. The body requires from 1 to 3 weeks to make the adaptation from being primarily a sugar burner to a fat burner. But once it does, performance levels return to normal and endurance gradually increases to new heights as an almost limitless supply of fat calories become readily available. Once the body has learned to use fat instead of exclusively glucose for energy, it becomes quicker and easier for the body to switch back and forth from sugar to fat burning.

Tim Noakes, MD, and colleagues at the Division of Exercise Science and Sports Medicine at the University of Cape Town have shown that dietary fat adaptation for a period of 2 to 4 weeks has resulted in a nearly twofold increase in resistance to fatigue during prolonged, low- to moderate-intensity cycling.[56]

Research at the University of Vermont found that a low-carb weight loss diet can improve athletic performance in untrained individuals. The researchers put overweight subjects on a calorie restricted, low-carb, high-fat diet for 6 weeks in a metabolic research ward. Treadmill performance testing of the subjects, which included a determination of peak aerobic power (VO_2max), was conducted at the beginning of the study and after 6 weeks on the diet. Endurance time to exhaustion was quantitated at 75 percent of the baseline VO_2max. This endurance test was repeated again after one week of weight loss and finally after 6 weeks of weight loss. Other than these tests, the subjects did no training exercise. During the study the subjects lost an average of more than 22 pounds (10 kg). The final endurance treadmill test was performed with the subjects carrying a backpack equivalent in weight to the amount lost. This way the subjects' exercise performance would not be influenced by their reduced body weight.

At the beginning of the study, average endurance time until exhaustion was 168 minutes. After one week, before the subjects' bodies had become fat adapted, time dropped to 130 minutes. But by the end of 6 weeks, the subjects were fully fat adapted and endurance time jumped to 249 minutes—an increase of 81 minutes, while carrying a backpack.[57]

The difference between highly trained athletes is not quite as dramatic but is still substantial. For this reason, many endurance athletes are switching to low-carb, high-fat diets, without calorie restriction, to enhance their performance.

PROTECTION FROM CHRONIC DISEASE

Eating fat, including saturated fat, doesn't shorten life, as we've often been told, but actually extends it. A growing body of evidence is showing that higher-fat diets increase lifespan. They do this by reducing the risk of chronic degenerative diseases such as heart disease, diabetes, Alzheimer's, and cancer, all of which are likely to send you to an early grave.

Fat has many important functions in the body. It helps regulate digestion and absorption of blood sugar, thus helping prevent insulin resistance and diabetes. Fat helps satisfy hunger longer, so you don't eat as often, thus helping you eat fewer calories. Therefore, eating fat helps you maintain proper weight. It supports normal hormone function, strengthens the immune system and helps ward off infections, helps maintain healthy digestive function, increases nutrient absorption for better nutrition, sharpens the mind, and energizes the body, all of which help support good health and avoid disease.

Despite what has been claimed about saturated fat and cardiovascular disease, fat actually protects against heart attacks and strokes. A study published in the *American Journal of Clinical Nutrition* in 2018 investigated the association of dairy fat with total mortality and cardiovascular disease among older adults. Dairy fat has often been criticized for its high saturated fat content. Nearly 3,000 adults age 65 years and older were included in the study, which measured plasma levels of fatty acids found in dairy fat. Unlike most previous studies, which relied on self-reported questionnaires, this study's measurement methodology provided a greater and more objective insight into the impact of long-term exposure to dairy fats.

The study found no significant link between dairy fats and cause of death or, more specifically, heart disease and strokes—two of our biggest killers. In fact, dairy fat was linked to lower cardiovascular disease deaths. People with higher fatty acid levels, suggesting higher consumption of whole-fat dairy, had a 42 percent lower risk of dying from stroke.[52] The results of this study were not unusual, many previous studies have also shown that the consumption of total fat, saturated fat, and unsaturated fat are associated with a reduced risk of ischemic stroke.[59-60] Ischemic stroke is caused by a blocked artery, the same process that causes heart attacks, and like heart attacks, is considered to be a consequence of atherosclerosis and cardiovascular disease. A study by Harvard researchers that measured atherosclerosis using angiography on 2,243 subjects over a 3-year period revealed that greater saturated fat intake was associated with *less* progression of coronary atherosclerosis, whereas carbohydrate intake was associated with a greater progression.[61] In addition, a greater saturated fat intake was associated with higher HDL cholesterol, higher apoprotein A-1, lower blood triglyceride levels, and lower triglyceride/HDL cholesterol ratio—all of which have been shown to reduce the risk of atherosclerosis and heart disease. These studies support recent meta-analyses that have shown that neither total fat nor saturated fat intake is associated with an increased risk of heart disease. These studies suggest that fat helps protect against heart disease and stroke.

This data is in agreement with the finding of a recent study conducted on a Dutch population involving 35,597 participants who were monitored for 12 years. Total saturated fat intake was found to be associated with a lower incidence of ischemic heart disease. Replacing saturated fats with animal protein, carbohydrate, and even unsaturated fats was found to significantly increase the risk of ischemic heart disease.[62]

In another recent study, diet and health data from subjects in 42 European countries was analyzed. Again, the researchers found no correlation between saturated fat intake and the incidence of heart disease. Instead, they found a link with high glycemic index foods—processed carbohydrates. The authors of the study called for a reassessment of government guidelines recommending restrictions on saturated fat consumption.[63]

In yet another study, researchers from McMaster University in Canada analyzed the associations of fat and carbohydrate intake with cardiovascular disease and mortality in 18 countries. The study involved 135,335 individuals 35 to 70 years of age, with a mean follow-up of 7.4 years. The primary outcomes were total deaths and major cardiovascular events (fatal cardiovascular disease, nonfatal heart attacks, stroke, and heart failure). The researchers assessed the associations between consumption of carbohydrate, total fat, and each type of fat with cardiovascular disease and death.

They found that high carbohydrate intake was associated with an increased incidence of death from all causes. In contrast, total fat, saturated fat, monounsaturated fat, and polyunsaturated fat were all associated with a lower risk of death, with no association with cardiovascular disease. Saturated fat intake was once again found to reduce the risk of stroke. This study showed that not eating enough fat could be harmful. People with the highest 20 percent in total fat intake (an average of 35.3 percent of calories from fat), had about a 23 percent reduced risk of death compared with the lowest 20 percent (an average of 10.6 percent of calories from fat).[64] Looking at the latest research reveals that in comparison to high-carb diets, high-fat diets are associated with less disease and a longer life.

9

Eat More Fat and
Fewer Carbs

A SUGAR EXPERIMENT

Australian filmmaker Damon Gameau wanted to know how much of an effect sugar actually has on our health. He decided to run an experiment on himself and find out. For the experiment he would eat a high-sugar, low-fat diet for 60 days. His journey would be documented on film and be monitored by a team of doctors and nutritionists.

Most of his life he ate a typical Western diet loaded with sugar and junk foods. For the previous three years, however; Gameau had been eating a low-carbohydrate, high-fat diet.

The average consumption of sugar in Australia, as well as most Western countries, is about 40 teaspoons per day. This is added sugar. It does not include the natural sugars found in fresh fruits and vegetables. It is the sugar that a person adds to his or her foods or that is added by food manufacturers.

We all know that eating too much sugar can be harmful. A diet filled with candy, soda, and desserts would be a disaster. Most people recognize this and try to eat what they believe are healthy foods. What is less obvious is that most of the foods sold in grocery stores contain hidden sugar—the sugar manufacturers add to their products. Eighty percent of all the foods sold in grocery stores contain added sugar.[1] For this reason, we consume far more sugar than we realize.

In this experiment, Gameau wasn't going to eat a diet loaded with candy and soda. His goal was to consume what was typical for the average Australian, 40 teaspoons of sugar a day. He would do this by eating only those foods that are perceived as being healthy. Foods on his list included such things as tomato soup, pork and beans, yogurt, fruit smoothies, granola breakfast cereal, muesli fruit and nut bars, and fruit juice. All foods, when

173

possible, were low-fat. These foods were supplemented by fresh meat and produce. He ate no candy or junk foods during the 60-day experiment.

In addition to the diet, Gameau was to maintain his normal exercise routine consisting of moderate running and strength training.

When he started the experiment he was concerned that he would have a difficult time reaching his 40 teaspoon limit each day. On his first day his breakfast consisted of a bowl of whole grain fruit and nut cereal, with a little yogurt, and a glass of apple juice. Total sugar content equaled 20 teaspoons. He was surprised at how much sugar was hidden in one meal. He soon discovered that consuming 40 teaspoons of sugar was easy even without any added sweets or pastries. The foods that supplied the greatest amount of hidden sugar were beverages, even the organic juices were loaded with sugar.

At the beginning of the experiment, Gameau was slender and in excellent health. He normally consumed about 2,300 calories a day: 50 percent of which consisted of fats from foods such as eggs and avocados, 26 percent consisted of protein from fish, chicken, and red meat, and 24 percent from carbohydrate, mostly fresh vegetables.

Gameau would eat poached eggs with avocado for breakfast, a salad sandwich and green smoothie for lunch, and some chicken and vegetables for dinner. During the experiment, however, he typically ate packaged cereal and low-fat yogurt for breakfast, a Subway sandwich and apple juice for lunch, and the same chicken and vegetables for dinner, but added a jar of Chicken Tonight or Teriyaki sauce to get his sugar count up for the day. He also started snacking on muesli bars and "healthy" fruit bars. He never used to snack, but the low-fat, high-carb diet increased his appetite, making it difficult for him to feel full and satiated.

When he started the new diet, Gameau weighed 167 pounds (76 kg), had a waist circumference of 33 inches (84 cm), low triglyceride levels, healthy liver function, and no signs of insulin resistance or diabetes.

After 60 days he was noticeably fatter, with a slightly protruding belly and a little more flesh hanging on his sides. In this short period of time he gained 19 pounds (8.6 kg) with an increase of 7 percent body fat. His waist circumference increased to 37 inches (94 cm)—a gain of 4 inches (10 cm). His triglyceride levels doubled, increasing his risk for heart disease. Liver enzymes in his blood indicated that he was developing fatty liver disease. His face was spotted with acne, which is often a sign of a toxic liver. Fasting blood glucose levels indicated he was developing insulin resistance. If he kept going with his new diet he was on his way to becoming obese and chronically sick.

Sugar companies insist that obesity is caused by eating too many calories and not getting enough exercise. In other words, we're fat because we are a bunch of lazy gluttons. Since 60 percent of the population is overweight, we must be a nation of sloths.

Throughout the experiment Gameau maintained his exercise routine, although as the experiment progressed, he found it increasingly difficult to keep up with it, primarily due to a lack of energy and enthusiasm. His physical activity level remained relatively constant throughout the 60 days, so his weight gain was not a result of inactivity.

Despite the fact that he gained a significant amount of weight and body fat and his waist circumference ballooned, he averaged about 2,300 calories a day—the same as he did before starting the experiment. If all calories are equal regardless of their source, as the sugar companies insist, he should not have gained any weight or body fat. Most of the calories he consumed before the experiment came from fat. During the experiment most of his calories came from sugar and other carbohydrates. In his case, it was obvious that all calories are not equal. Fat calories do not equal carbohydrate calories. The latter had a much greater effect on fat storage as well as shifting all health markers in an unhealthy direction.

The most surprising effect Gameau experienced wasn't physical but was psychological. The diet affected his cognition, mood, and ability to concentrate. When he ate sugar, a childish side with a manic edge to it, came out. After awhile he would feel vague and aloof. Before breakfast, he felt exhausted just waiting for his morning sugar fix. As soon as he ate breakfast, he would feel wired from the sugar rush. After about an hour, he would crash and stay that way until he could get his next sugar fix. His girlfriend described him as uncharacteristically moody during the experiment. He noticed the mood swings at first, but in time became less aware of them as they became a regular part of his daily experience.

As soon as the experiment ended, Gameau resumed his normal no-sugar diet. During the first few weeks without sugar he went through a period of withdrawal. He had headaches, slept poorly, and was easily irritated. The first thing in the morning he craved sugar. These effects gradually wore off and after 2 months without sugar his skin cleared up, his moods stabilized, he slept better, he lost 13 pounds (6 kg), and his blood tests returned to normal.

Gameau's experience illustrates what is happening to all of us who eat a typical "healthy" Western diet. Although we may believe we are making wise dietary choices, if those foods are loaded with hidden sugar, as most are, they are tearing down your health. It is no wonder obesity, diabetes, Alzheimer's, and other chronic diseases are epidemic.

Gameau's experiment was filmed and made into a documentary titled *That Sugar Film*. It is worth watching.

MISGUIDED GUIDELINE

The dietary advice that is generally advocated internationally is patterned after the *Dietary Guidelines for Americans*, which was first published jointly in 1980 by the US Department of Agriculture (USDA) and the US Department of Health and Human Services (HHS). These guidelines serve as the foundation for all federal nutrition recommendations and education activities. Beginning with the 1985 edition, the USDA and HHS appointed a Dietary Guidelines Advisory Committee of nutrition and health experts to review and update the guidelines every 5 years. All of the editions of the *Dietary Guidelines* have recommended a diet that is low in fat and saturated fat, with later editions recommending reducing saturated fat to less than 10 percent of total calories. It further recommends that total carbohydrate intake be increased to form the foundation of a healthy diet. Initially there was no limitation placed on refined carbohydrates, although there was a weak suggestion to reduce added sugar consumption.

These guidelines are based on the cholesterol hypothesis that was first proposed by Ancel Keys in the 1950s. The hypothesis led to the general belief that eating food rich in saturated fat and cholesterol increased blood cholesterol, and therefore, must increase the risk of heart disease. In addition, it was believed that since fat is more calorie dense than carbohydrate or protein, a reduction in its consumption would lead to a reduction in calories and a decrease in the incidence of obesity, as well as diabetes and other dietary related disorders.

Since 1980 the low-fat diet, in its various forms, has been touted as the optimal way to eat and has been recommended as the go-to diet for weight loss, diabetes care, and the prevention of cardiovascular disease, as well as just about every other health issue imaginable. Saturated fat more than any other type of fat has been pegged as the principal troublemaker—the root cause of obesity and heart disease and a contributor to just about every other ailment of modern society.

The American Heart Association (and others) recommends that we limit our fat intake to 30 percent or less of total calories, down from the 40 percent we had been consuming before the *Guidelines for Americans*. Some doctors recommended we lower it even more, to 20 percent or less. The idea that fat was unhealthy became firmly established in the public's mind. In the 1980s, food manufacturers, sensitive to customers' growing desire to avoid fats, began to produce a wide variety of nonfat and low-fat foods. As total fat in the diet decreased, it was replaced with an increased amount of carbohydrate. Protein-rich foods, such as meat, eggs, and cheese, were also generally high in fat, so people did not increase their consumption of these types of foods, and protein consumption remained fairly consistent. A low-fat diet, consequently, became a high-carb diet. When people started eating more carbohydrate, they didn't increase the amount of high-fiber foods, such as vegetables or whole grains, but increased their intake of processed, refined starches and sugars. Adding more vegetables into the diet would likely not have been a problem, but replacing fats with refined carbs has been a dietary disaster. As a result, obesity and chronic disease have skyrocketed.

According to a statistical review of dietary data published in the journal *Nutrition*, following the advice given in the *Dietary Guidelines for Americans*, consumption of fats in the United States has dropped 11 percent, with a corresponding increase in carbohydrate consumption of 12 percent of total caloric intake. From 1971 to 2011 average weight and body mass index have increased dramatically, with the percentage of overweight or obese Americans increasing from 42 percent in 1971 to over 66 percent in 2011.[2] By 2015 that number had risen to 73 percent. This rise in obesity has been followed by an epidemic of diabetes, Alzheimer's, and other metabolic syndrome related disorders.[3]

Since the introduction of the low-fat, high-carbohydrate dietary recommendations, there has been a dramatic acceleration in the prevalence of chronic diseases and disorders. Many conditions that are known to be associated with or exacerbated by sugar and refined starch have more than doubled since 1990. In the United States, over the course of a single generation (25 years) from 1990 to 2015, these conditions, among many others, have increased dramatically, as shown in the following table:

Condition	Percent Increase	
Multiple sclerosis	117	
Inflammatory bowel disease	120	**Increase in Chronic**
ADHD	139	**Disease from 1990-2015**
Asthma	142	
COPD	148	
Obesity	260	
Stroke	262	
Depression	280	
Alzheimer's	299	
Diabetes	305	
Sleep apnea	430	
Osteoarthritis	449	Source: Richard Lear
Cataracts	480	"The Root Cause in the
Hypothyroidism	702	Dramatic Rise of Chronic
Fibromyalgia	7,727	Disease," https://app.box.
Bipolar disease in youth	10,833	com/s/iyjuzrxtkx3gpblu-
Chronic fatigue syndrome	11,027	4vmt0wjrgsxykuzc.

177

The dramatic increase in the prevalence of these conditions is obviously not due to genetics, because it is impossible for genetic disorders to increase like this over a single generation. This is the pattern of a plague—something in the environment or diet is the cause. The most obvious change during this period has been our diet.

This isn't just an American problem. Most nations have adopted similar dietary guidelines, avoiding fat in favor of more carbohydrate, and consequently, are also suffering from an obesity epidemic and health crisis. According to the World Health Organization, worldwide obesity has nearly tripled since 1975. In 2016, 39 percent of adults aged 18 years and over were overweight, and 13 percent were obese. As in the United States, the incidence of chronic disease is skyrocketing.

LOW-FAT VERSUS LOW-CARB DIETS

Early on, some doctors challenged the low-fat paradigm. The most influential, perhaps, was Robert Atkins, MD. Atkins was a cardiologist who realized that the low-fat dietary approach to weight loss didn't work and that a low-carb diet was much more effective. Not only was a low-carb diet more successful in helping people lose excess weight, but patients' overall health improved dramatically. His program focused on limiting total carbohydrate intake, with no restriction on protein or fat. Consequently, his diet was often high in total fat and saturated fat. In fact, the first couple of weeks of his diet limited total carbohydrate intake to just 20 grams per day, with a significant increase in fat. To the dismay of doctors and dietitians everywhere, those who followed his plan lost weight easily and quickly even though they had previously failed miserably with the standard low-fat weight reducing diets. Doctors warned that such a high-fat diet would eventually increase blood pressure, raise cholesterol levels, clog arteries, and lead to an early death from cardiovascular disease. Just the opposite happened. Signs and symptoms of heart disease dramatically improved, people felt better, had more energy, and various other health problems vanished. The success of Atkins's diet grew in popularity and his book *Dr. Atkins' New Diet Revolution* became a bestseller. The positive results that thousands of people experienced with the Atkins diet instilled doubt in the minds of many, including doctors, about the low-fat approach to weight loss and better health.

Researchers bent on discrediting low-carb diets began doing studies comparing the results to low-fat diets. The researchers must have been mystified and perhaps even outraged by the results. In every case where a fair comparison was made, the low-carb diet came out the winner. Some researchers tried to trivialize the results by saying the difference was insignificant and claimed that following a low-carb diet would lead to heart disease, but when they also measured cardiovascular parameters, such as blood pressure and cholesterol levels, the low-carb dieters' numbers were significantly improved.

In an attempt to learn which of all the popular diets at the time was the most beneficial, researchers at Stanford University Medical School designed a yearlong head-to-head study between the Atkins diet and the Zone, Ornish, and LEARN diets. The Zone diet advocates a relatively balanced diet of 30 percent fat, 30 percent protein, and 40 percent carbohydrate. The LEARN (Lifestyle, Exercise, Attitudes, Relationships, and Nutrition) diet follows the American government's recommendations for a diet low in fat and high in carbohydrate, along with several lifestyle changes. The Ornish diet also involves lifestyle changes as well as calorie restriction and very low-fat intake. The study was published in the *Journal of the American Medical Association* in 2007.

At the end of the yearlong study, the Atkins diet came out the clear winner in both weight loss and overall improvement in measurable health parameters, such as cholesterol and blood glucose levels. Subjects on the Atkins diet lost more than twice as much weight as any of the other diets with no signs of undesirable side effects. Those in the Atkins group achieved greater reductions in weight, body fat, triglycerides, and blood pressures, and a greater increase in HDL cholesterol—all signs of improved cardio-vascular and overall health.[4]

Any way you look at it, the Atkins diet performed better than all these other popular diets. "This is the best study so far to compare popular diets," said Walter Willett, chair of the department of nutrition of the Harvard School of Public Health. The findings confirm, he said, that reducing carbohydrates, "especially those with refined starch and sugar like that found in the US diet, has metabolic benefits." It also shows that replacing carbohydrates with fat "can improve blood cholesterol fractions and blood pressure."

These results were reconfirmed by another team of investigators in a randomized, controlled, dietary intervention trial published the following year. This study compared a low-fat diet, containing less than 10 percent saturated fat, to a low-carbohydrate diet, with 12 percent of total calories from carbohydrate.[5]

Both diets in this study were low in calories (1,500/day); however, the low-carb diet showed greater improvements in numerous health markers, including lower abdominal fat and body mass index, blood lipid levels (tri-glycerides, apolipoprotein B), glucose tolerance (blood glucose, insulin, and insulin resistance), inflammation (tumor necrosis factor alpha, interleukin (IL) 6, IL-8, monocyte chemotactic protein 1, E-selectin, intercellular adhesion molecule 1), and risk factors for atherosclerosis (plasminogen activator inhibitor 1). In addition, the low-carb diet increased HDL, reduced ApoB/ApoA-1 ratio, and reduced small dense LDL. Overall, the low-carb diet showed a much greater improvement in health markers and reduced risk of cardiovascular and metabolic disease.

Some researchers wondered if reducing fat, as well as foods high in refined starch and sugar, without actually reducing other carbohydrates would produce similar or better results than a low-carb diet. Researchers at Duke University decided to find out by comparing a low-glycemic index diet to a low-carb, high-fat diet. The study involved 84 obese, type 2 diabetic subjects. In this study, subjects eating the low-fat, low glycemic index diet also reduced their total calorie intake by 500 calories per day. Although calorie intake was reduced and high glycemic index foods limited, carbohydrate intake still accounted for about 55 percent of total calories consumed. Those eating the low-carb, high-fat diet, had no calorie restriction and ate as much as they wanted. The main objective of the study was to compare blood sugar control in diabetic subjects. After 24 weeks, both diets led to improvements in the parameters measured. However, the low-carb, high-fat diet produced the best results: blood sugar, determined by A1C levels, was reduced 1.5 percent vs 0.5 percent; weight loss (without purposely reducing calorie intake) was greater 24.5 pounds (11.1 kg) vs 15.2 pounds (6.9 kg); and greater reduction in risk against heart disease was evidenced by an increase in HDL of 5.6 mg/dl vs 0 mg/dl. Both diets led to improvements in blood sugar control resulting in a reduction in diabetic medications taken. Those on the low-carb, high-fat diet reduced or eliminated diabetic medications by 95.2 percent compared to 62 percent in the low glycemic index diet group. Many other health markers such as blood pressure, and triglycerides also improved, but the differences between the groups were not statistically significant.[6] Although the reduction in sugar, refined starch, and total calories in the low glycemic index diet improved health markers, reducing total carbohydrate and increasing fat intake produced substantially better results.

Many additional studies have been published over the past few years, and virtually all of them have verified that low-carb, high-fat diets produce greater weight loss, better blood cholesterol and triglyceride levels, better blood sugar control, and lower markers for inflammation than low-fat diets.[7-15]

The scientific community in general now recognizes low-carbohydrate diets as superior to low-fat diets. However, despite the evidence, many medical professionals, organizations, and government agencies continue to support and promote low-fat dieting for philosophical (e.g., vegetarianism) or monetary reasons.

LIVE LONG AND HEALTHY WITH FEWER CARBS AND MORE FAT

Removing fat in the diet and replacing it with carbohydrate has proven to be a huge mistake that has led us down the path of obesity and diabetes. From a scientific point of view this makes sense. It is carbohydrate that affects blood sugar and insulin levels that lead to weight gain and metabolic dysfunction, not fat. Fat is an essential nutrient that is required for multiple purposes, as explained in the previous chapter. We have essential and conditionally essential fatty acids that are absolutely required in our diet. Fatty acids are needed for many purposes ranging from structural components for cell membranes to achieving and maintaining metabolic homeostasis. In contrast, the only purpose for dietary carbohydrate is as a source of fuel. There is no such thing as an essential carbohydrate. We do not require carbohydrate in our diet. This is amply demonstrated by the many meat-eating populations who, after weaning, consume no carbohydrate at all for the rest of their lives. Fat and protein can provide all the energy the body needs.

Many people are now recognizing that fats, including saturated fats, are not as bad as once believed and that we can add fats back into our diets without undue fear. Some acknowledge that low-carb diets can be beneficial and even superior to low-fat diets. Many doctors and dietitians admit that a healthy diet can include fat, yet may still add the caveat, "But don't eat too much." How much is too much? Should we follow the recommendation in the *Guidelines for Americans* and limit our total fat intake to no more than 30 percent of total calories? Or can we eat as much as our grandparents and great-grandparents used to eat and what the average consumption was before the *Guidelines* were issued and go back to eating 40 to 45 percent of calories as fat? Or could we perhaps even increase our fat intake to that of certain traditional populations, like the Inuit, that consumed as much as 85 to 90 percent of their calories as fat? Why limit fat consumption at all? Is there any harm in eating a very high-fat diet? It apparently did not hurt the Inuit and other hunter-gatherer cultures. They certainly did not suffer from obesity, diabetes, metabolic syndrome, or any of the degenerative diseases we are plagued with in our high-carbohydrate society.

Recognizing that carbohydrates, principally refined carbohydrates and sugar, are the real cause of most of our health problems, it might be reasoned that reducing total carbohydrate intake or eliminating refined carbohydrate and sugar would greatly improve health. Studies have clearly shown that low-carb diets, which generally also happen to be higher-fat diets, promote better health than low-fat diets. Historical evidence from hunter-gatherer populations also shows that very high-fat diets are superior to our typical high-carb diet. It is apparent that even very high-fat diets are not harmful and might be beneficial, perhaps even therapeutic.

WHAT IS A LOW-CARB DIET?

There is no official definition of a low-carbohydrate diet. However, a diet that is limited to 100 grams of carbohydrate or less a day is generally considered low-carb. On average, most people consume between 200 and 300 grams of carbohydrate a day, mostly from refined grains, starchy vegetables, sugary beverages, and sweets. Many people eat much more. Consuming 300 grams of carbohydrate in a day isn't difficult. Consider that one regular size plain bagel contains 53 grams of carbs, a slice of white bread 13 grams, a 12 ounce soda 37 grams, and a 6-inch bean and cheese burrito 33 grams. Let's look at how many carbs a person might consume in a day.

Breakfast: 6 pancakes (4 inches/10 cm diameter) with syrup, 180 grams; plus a small glass (8 oz/227 g) of fresh squeezed orange juice, 25 grams. Meal total 205 grams of carbs.

Lunch: 1 regular size hamburger with catsup, 25 grams; small fries (2.5 ounces/71 g) 22 grams; and a 12 ounce soda, 37 grams. Meal total 84 grams of carbs.

Dinner: 2 cups spaghetti with tomato sauce and meat, 92 grams; 2 slices of garlic toast, 26 grams; and a small tossed salad (1 cup/84 g) with oil and vinegar dressing, 4 grams. Meal total 122 grams.

The total amount of carbohydrate for the day comes to 386 grams. Keep in mind this is without any dessert, candy, or snacks, and the portion sizes mentioned were modest.

A basic low-carb diet focuses on restricting only the amount and type of carbohydrate eaten without any special restriction on protein or fat. Since grains, starchy vegetables (e.g., potatoes, legumes), and sweets contain the highest percentage of carbohydrate, they are generally eliminated or at least severely restricted. Many fruits, especially dried fruit, contain a high amount of sugar, so they must also be limited.

Foods that are low in carbohydrate and make up the bulk of a low-carb diet include meats, fish, eggs, unsweetened dairy, nuts and seeds, non-starchy vegetables, and occasionally some fruits. A low-carb diet can encompass a wide range of dietary preferences. It can be protein based, supplemented with vegetables, or be vegetable based, accompanied by a modest amount of meat and dairy. Fat intake can be modest or heavy. Considering the importance of having an adequate amount of fat in the diet and the fact that fat is not harmful, fat should contribute a significant amount of the calories.

10

The Ketogenic Diet

MORE THAN JUST A MEANS FOR WEIGHT LOSS

By definition, the ketogenic diet is one that is very low in carbohydrate, very high in fat, with moderate protein. In contrast to a typical low-carb diet, the ketogenic diet generally has fewer carbs and more fat and limits protein intake. It is not a high-protein diet, as many low-carb diets are. The reduction in carbohydrate (mostly starch and sugar) and the addition of good fats can produce remarkable therapeutic effects. Although the diet is most commonly thought of as a weight loss diet, it was originally developed as a treatment for epilepsy.

In the early 1900s fasting therapy was a popular form of treatment for chronic or serious conditions such as cancer, arthritis, and digestive problems. Epilepsy responded very well to fasting therapy and significantly reduced the severity and frequency of seizures, with results that would last for months or years. Patients were routinely put on water only fasts for 2 to 3 weeks or more. Doctors noticed that the longer they could keep a patient on a fast, the better the outcome. However, there was a limit on the amount of time a patient could endure a water only fast. So, doctors developed a diet that could mimic the metabolic and therapeutic effects of fasting but allow the patient enough nutrients to maintain good health over an extended period. This became known as the ketogenic diet.

When fasting, no carbohydrate is consumed, so blood sugar and insulin levels remain low, but normal. The body always maintains a certain minimum level of blood sugar even during a fast. If no carbohydrate is eaten, then body protein is converted into glucose to maintain blood glucose levels and stored fat is used as the main source of energy. Despite not consuming any calories, vitamins, or minerals, patients improved.

Since dietary fat and protein do not significantly affect blood glucose or insulin levels, it was reasoned that eliminating carbohydrate from the diet could mimic the metabolic effects of fasting, and hopefully also the therapeutic effects as well. The ketogenic diet was first tested on epileptic patients in 1921 with remarkable success. The diet proved just as successful as fasting, but now patients could eat foods and maintain the diet for months or even years. As the time on the diet increased, so did the success rate. Doctors were seeing dramatic reductions in seizure activity and even complete lifelong cures to a disease that was once considered incurable. Over time, it was discovered that most patients could permanently reduce seizure activity by 90 to 100 percent after eating a ketogenic diet for a period of 2 years, after which they gradually transitioned back to eating an ordinary diet. This amount of time allowed the brain to rewire and heal itself.

The success seen with epilepsy and the improvement seen in health markers that doctors use to evaluate a patient's health, led researchers to investigate the effects of the ketogenic diet on other neurological disorders such as Alzheimer's, Parkinson's, autism, ALS, stroke, traumatic brain injury, multiple sclerosis, migraine headaches, depression, and even various forms of brain cancer.[1-12]

In every case, the diet proved highly successful in easing the symptoms and in some cases restoring normal or near normal function.

Chronic inflammation leads to insulin resistance. When that inflammation is in the brain, it can cause brain insulin resistance. Insulin resistance is the hallmark feature of type 2 diabetes. Alzheimer's disease, as stated earlier in this book, has recently been identified as a form of diabetes and is now referred to as type 3 diabetes—diabetes of the brain. Brain cells use glucose as their primary source of fuel. However, insulin resistance interferes with glucose metabolism, making it difficult for the brain cells to absorb glucose. Consequently, the affected part of the brain becomes starved of energy and begins to degenerate and die. As the brain shrinks, memory fades, cognitive skills are lost, and even personality changes. As noted earlier, fatty acids cannot fulfill the brain's energy needs, and therefore requires an alternative energy source—ketones. Ketones are not affected by insulin resistance. Brain cells can quickly and easily absorb ketones even in a state of insulin resistance, providing the energy the brain cells need to live and carry out their intended functions. This can help prevent brain degeneration. All brain disorders are accompanied by chronic inflammation, interfering with normal glucose metabolism. This is why the ketogenic diet has shown to be effective in treating various brains disorders. As noted in previous chapters, sugar promotes inflammation and destroys the brain, while fats (ketones) heal it.

The original ketogenic diet was severe, limiting carbohydrate intake to just 2 percent of total calories with the consumption of 90 percent fat and 8 percent protein. Every meal and every snack had to have these exact proportions of nutrients. Parents of epileptic children had to take special cooking classes to learn how to prepare meals properly. As you might imagine, meals consisting of 90 percent fat and only 2 carbohydrate were not generally appealing. Many patients could not tolerate the diet, and parents usually had to prepare two meals, one for the patient and the other for the rest of the family. Most families opted for medications rather than endure the diet even though the diet may only be required for a year or two.

When we do not consume any carbohydrate for a period of time, such as between meals, while sleeping during the night, or when fasting, blood glucose levels decline. Our cells, however, work and function tirelessly 24 hours a day and consequently, require a continual source of energy. As blood glucose levels fall, fatty acids are pulled out of storage from our fat cells to supply the needed energy. In this manner, our cells always have access to either glucose or fatty acids to supply their energy needs.

This process works very well for the body, but not for the brain. The brain can use glucose but it cannot use fatty acids to fulfill its energy needs, and therefore relies on ketones as an alternative source of energy. When blood glucose levels fall, the liver converts fatty acids into ketones. Most of the cells in the body can use ketones as fuel, but they are essential for the brain when glucose becomes less available.

Over time, it was discovered that restricting carbohydrate to just 2 percent of total calories was not necessary to achieve a state of ketosis—when fatty acids and ketones supply most of the body's energy needs. When ketosis is brought about by manipulating the diet, it is often referred to as *nutritional ketosis*. Most people can get into mild nutritional ketosis by restricting their total carbohydrate intake to 40 or 50 grams per day. Moderate ketosis is generally achieved with a carbohydrate restriction of about 30 grams and high ketosis with a restriction of fewer than 20 grams.

It was also discovered that it was not necessary to consume 90 percent of calories as fat. A more manageable ketogenic diet could be achieved by reducing total fat intake to about 60 percent of calories and increasing carbohydrate and protein intake accordingly. This made the diet far more palatable and easier to manage.

When in ketosis, the body burns its stored fat to produce energy; consequently, many people following the diet lost weight and did so easily. An added benefit was that ketosis depresses feelings of hunger, so people can cut down on the number of calories they consume while still eating to satisfaction, further enhancing the weight loss effects. The initial stage of Dr. Atkins's diet, which limited carbohydrate intake to 20 grams or less, shifted people into a state of nutritional ketosis. The results were impressive.

Consequently, the ketogenic diet shifted from being just a treatment for epilepsy to also being an effective treatment for weight loss.

THE KETOGENIC DIET IMPROVES ALL HEALTH MARKERS

In the 1990s low-carb and ketogenic diets started to become a popular means for weight loss. Doctors leery of how a very high-fat diet might affect their patients' health, kept a close eye on how the diet affected health markers such as blood pressure and lipid levels. Physicians and dietitians were surprised to find that the ketogenic diet improved all of the common parameters doctors measure to evaluate a person's health status and risk for disease.

For years the standard medically approved diet given to patients to improve their health or to lose excess weight was the low-fat, calorie-restricted diet. The ketogenic diet is essentially the opposite—high in fat and eating to satisfaction.

Despite the fact that patients were experiencing remarkable improvements in their health, the ketogenic diet remained controversial. Many doctors and researchers just couldn't believe that a high-fat diet could be healthy. This led investigators to compare the effects of the ketogenic diet with the standard low-fat diet in clinical trials.

For example, researchers at the University of Connecticut compared cardiovascular risk factors of two groups of overweight men, one following a very low-carb, high-fat diet and the other following a low-fat, low-calorie diet. Blood tests were performed at the beginning of the study and at its conclusion 6 weeks later. Both diets showed improvements in total blood cholesterol levels, blood insulin levels, and insulin resistance, but the differences in these parameters between the two groups were not significant, which demonstrated that the high-fat diet is just as good as a low-fat diet. However, only the low-carb, high-fat group had significantly lower fasting triglycerides, triglyceride/HDL ratio, and blood glucose levels, which showed the superiority of the ketogenic diet.

The ketogenic group also had better LDL cholesterol readings. LDL cholesterol is often referred to as the "bad cholesterol" because it is believed to be the primary type of cholesterol that leaves deposits in the arteries. However, as you have learned from a previous chapter, there are two types of LDL cholesterol: one large and buoyant and the other small and dense. The large, buoyant LDL is harmless, in fact, it is actually beneficial because it is the type of cholesterol that is incorporated into cell membranes to give them strength, and is also used to produce vitamin D and many of our hormones, such as testosterone and estrogen. It is the small, dense LDL cholesterol

186

that is associated with oxidation and increased risk of heart disease. Blood tests generally do not separate the two and only give a single value for the total. The number for total LDL is thus completely useless. In this study, the two types of LDL were measured separately. Total LDL cholesterol was significantly reduced by the low-fat diet but not by the low-carb diet. On the surface this may appear to show an advantage to the low-fat diet, but that is not the case. While the total LDL did not change much in the low-carb diet, the type of LDL did, decreasing the undesirable small LDL and increasing the beneficial large LDL. Although the low-fat diet decreased total LDL, it did not significantly improve the percentage of the good LDL.[13]

In addition to the better blood lipid and sugar levels, the ketogenic group also lost significantly more weight: 13.5 pounds (6.1 kg) versus 8.6 pounds (3.9 kg). All these changes indicate a much greater reduction in the risk of heart disease and diabetes in comparison to a low-fat diet.

Researchers at Duke University performed a similar study.[14] One hundred twenty overweight, hyperlipidemic (i.e., those with high cholesterol) men and women volunteered for the study. Half of the subjects ate a ketogenic diet (fewer than 20 grams of carbohydrate per day) with no calorie limit; they could eat as much meat, fat, and eggs as they wanted. The other half ate a low-fat, low-cholesterol, calorie-restricted diet (reduced by 500–1,000 calories per day).

After 24 weeks, the low-fat group lost 10.6 pounds (4.8 kg) of body fat, while the ketogenic group lost 20.7 pounds (9.4 kg), twice as much as the low-fat group. For weight loss, this study clearly demonstrated the advantage of the ketogenic diet. Blood pressure, which had been slightly elevated in the test subjects at the beginning of the study, decreased in both groups. In the low-fat group, systolic (top number) and diastolic (bottom number) blood pressure decreased by 7.5 and 5.2 mm Hg, respectively. In the ketogenic group, systolic and diastolic blood pressure decreased by 9.6 and 6.0 mm Hg, respectively. The higher your blood pressure is, the greater your risk of heart disease. Even a small increase in blood pressure increases risk. The advantage again went to the ketogenic group.

Blood triglycerides are considered an independent and separate risk factor from cholesterol for heart disease; the higher the triglyceride level, the greater the risk. Blood triglyceride levels dropped by 27.9 mg/dl (0.32 mmol/l) in the low-fat group but fell by a whopping 74.2 mg/dl (0.83 mmol/l) in the ketogenic group, more than 2.5 times as much as the low-fat group. HDL cholesterol is considered the "good" cholesterol and is believed to help protect against heart disease; the higher this number, the better. HDL cholesterol *decreased* by 1.6 mg/dl (0.041 mmol/l) in the low-fat group but increased by 5.5 mg/dl (0.142 mmol/l) in the ketogenic group.

The cholesterol ratio (total cholesterol/HDL) is considered far more accurate as an indicator of heart disease risk in comparison to total cholesterol or LDL values. The lower the ratio, the lower the risk. The cholesterol ratio dropped by 0.3 in the low-fat group and by 0.6 in the ketogenic group, twice that of the low-fat group.

Another independent risk factor is the triglyceride/HDL ratio. The smaller the ratio, the better. The low-fat group saw a drop of 0.6, while the ketogenic group fell by 1.6, or nearly three times as much. The triglyceride/HDL ratio is considered one of the most accurate indicators of heart disease risk. A ratio of 6 or more indicates very high risk, a ratio of 4 or more signals high risk, and a ratio of 2 or less is ideal, or low risk. At the end of the study, the low-fat group's ratio averaged 3.4, indicating moderate risk, while the ketogenic group averaged 1.6, signifying very low risk of heart disease. With each risk factor measured, the ketogenic diet proved superior to the low-fat diet, collaborating the results of the previously mentioned study.

A number of additional studies have compared these two diets, and in every case the high-fat or ketogenic diet has proven superior at improving standard health markers.[15-21] Even in long-term studies lasting up to 2 years, the results have been the same.[22] High-fat, ketogenic diets have proven to be not only safe, but more effective at improving overall health and reducing the risk of chronic disease than low-fat diets.

In comparison to low-fat diets, the ketogenic diet shows superior results with the following health markers:

- reduces blood glucose/A1C (improves insulin sensitivity)
- reduces blood insulin
- raises HDL
- reduces blood triglycerides
- increases large, beneficial LDL
- reduces small, dense LDL
- reduces body weight and BMI (fat loss)
- reduces waist circumference (visceral fat loss)
- normalizes blood pressure
- reduces cholesterol ratio (total cholesterol/HDL)
- reduces triglyceride ratio (triglyceride/HDL)
- reduces C-reactive protein (lower systemic inflammation)
- increases human growth hormone levels (HGH)
- reduces AGEs
- reduces oxidative stress

In addition to improving common health markers, those who follow a ketogenic diet often experience improved mental clarity and sharper memory, have more energy, sleep more soundly, have better digestive function, gain relief from aches and pains associated with inflammation, break free from sugar addictions and uncontrollable food cravings, are happier, and enjoy an overall improvement in physical and mental health.

The improvement in health with a low-carb, high-fat diet eliminates the need for medications. One of the remarkable things about this diet is that it corrects so many metabolic defects that you will be able to reduce or discontinue many of the medications you may be taking. You may also feel an immediate improvement as soon as you discontinue them since you won't be burdened with the unpleasant side effects that often accompany drug treatment.

The diet improves blood lipid levels, eliminating the purpose for cholesterol medication. It balances blood sugar and insulin, so diabetic medications and insulin become unnecessary. Even type 1 diabetics who cannot produce normal amounts of insulin can lower and possibly eliminate insulin injections. High blood pressure will come down naturally. Hormone levels balance out. Systemic inflammation calms down. Chronic headaches go away. Mood and energy levels improve, eliminating the need for antidepressants. Anyone going on a ketogenic diet should have his or her doctor monitor medication use and reduce them as needed.

THE THERAPEUTIC EFFECTS OF KETONES

Ketones are derived from fatty acids. Like fatty acids, they can be used by our cells as a source of fuel to power our cells, but they are far more than just a source of energy. Once believed to be simply fragments of partially metabolized fatty acids, they are now recognized as specialized molecules with numerous important functions.

The primary function of ketones is to serve as an alternative fuel, especially for the brain. Ketones are compact sources of fuel that deliver more energy than glucose. For this reason, they are often referred to as the brain's superfuel. They increase energy production by 25 percent in comparison to glucose while reducing oxygen consumption.

Unlike glucose or fatty acids, ketones do not require insulin to enter the cell and pass into the mitochondria, where they are converted into energy. This is especially critical for cells that are crippled by desensitization to insulin (e.g., insulin resistance). Insulin is necessary to shuttle glucose into the cells, but no insulin is needed to allow ketones to enter. This can supply insulin-resistant cells with a boost of life-giving energy.

One of the unfortunate consequences of converting glucose into energy is the production of destructive free radicals. It is like the exhaust expelled when a car engine burns gasoline. In the case of our cells, the exhaust is free radicals. Healthy, well-nourished cells, however, are prepared for this and carry with them a reserve of protective antioxidants that neutralize the free radicals, reducing the damage they may cause. When ketones are used to produce energy in place of glucose, much less oxygen is needed, which greatly reduces the formation of free radicals and conserves precious antioxidants. Ketones essentially act like a high-grade, clean-burning, high-potency fuel that produces little exhaust and gives more power. In people with chronic health problems, antioxidant reserves are so depleted that free radicals generated from various sources run wild, promoting inflammation and degeneration.[23]

Ketones also reduce oxidative stress caused by AGEs—the destructive molecules that promote premature aging and disease. High-carb diets raise blood glucose levels, increasing the formation of AGEs. The ketogenic diet keeps blood glucose levels low, decreasing the production of AGEs and their accompanying free radicals. In addition, ketones alter gene expression, causing cells to increase their production of protective antioxidant enzymes such as catalase, glutathione, glutathione peroxidase, and superoxide dismutase.[24] Ketones also stimulate the production of the antioxidant metallothionein, which is believed to provide protection against oxidative stress and heavy metal toxicity.[25] Reducing oxidative stress in cells and tissues is one of the major reasons for the anti-aging effects observed from the ketogenic diet.

Almost every disease involves runaway inflammation and poor oxygen and glucose utilization. Ketones improve oxygen utilization and calm inflammation, thereby potentially providing protection against a large number of disease conditions.

Ketones provide the cells with a quick and potent source of energy, requiring less oxygen and producing far fewer free radicals in the process. Cells get the boost of energy they need to meet their energy demands to function as they were meant to. Protective antioxidant levels remain high, and the cells work at a heightened level of efficiency. Brain and nerve cells function better, heart cells become more efficient, and in fact, all the cells in the body that use ketones work better. Efficiency improves. For example, ketones improve the function and efficiency of the heart muscle, increasing hydraulic output by 28 percent.[26] Certain health-promoting genes are activated, and genes that promote inflammation and ill health are deactivated.

Ketones have traditionally been viewed as solely an alternative fuel to glucose. However, ketones themselves possess potent health-promoting effects independent of carbohydrate restriction and many of the beneficial effects associated with the ketogenic diet are, at least in part, due to them.

Ketone ester supplements have been used in research to increase blood ketone levels, without the need of going on a ketogenic diet. It appears that ketones can independently lower both blood glucose and insulin levels. In a study with mice, when 30 percent of the dietary calories from starch was replaced with ketone esters, blood glucose decreased by about 50 percent, from 5 to 2.8 mmol/l, and insulin decreased from 0.54 to 0.26 mg/ml.[27] Insulin sensitivity is increased (e.g., insulin resistance is decreased). Ketones have the ability to mimic some of the effects of insulin.[28]

Ketones have shown to reduce inflammation and oxidative stress and can reduce the detrimental effects of hypoxia (oxygen deficiency).[29-30] Oxygen is vital for proper brain function. The brain depends on oxygen so much that although it represents only 2 percent of the mass of the body, it consumes some 20 percent of the oxygen. Consequently, brain cells are extremely sensitive to oxygen deprivation. Without oxygen, some brain cells start dying in less than five minutes, leading to brain damage or death. Hypoxia can be caused by asphyxiation, carbon monoxide poisoning, cardiac arrest (heart attack), choking, drowning, strangulation, stroke, very low blood pressure, and drug overdose. Ketones block the detrimental effects of hypoxia by improving oxygen delivery. In a study where ketones were administered intravenously, raising blood ketone levels to 2.16 mmol/l (the level of about a 3 day-fast), blood flow to the brain increased by 39 percent, improving circulation and oxygen availability.[31] A number of studies show that ketones protect the brain against the damage caused by the interruption of oxygen delivery to the brain.[32-34]

Ketones stimulate the activity of brain-derived neurotrophic factors (BDNF)—small proteins that exert protective and nourishing actions on neurons.[35] These proteins play a crucial role in neuron survival and function. Neurotrophic factors regulate the growth of neurons, associated metabolic functions such as protein synthesis, and the ability of the neuron to make neurotransmitters that carry the chemical signals that allow neurons to communicate with each other.

Ketones also supply the lipid building blocks needed to grow new neurons.[36] Thus, they aid in the regrowth or repair of damaged brain cells and the synthesis of new cells. This is exciting because it means that ketones potentially provide a means to reverse much of the damage caused by a number of neurological disorders.

Disturbance in glucose metabolism is an underlying problem common in most neurodegenerative diseases. Ketones provide an alternative—and more effective—source of energy that bypasses the defect in glucose metabolism giving the neurons the life-giving energy they need to function properly and provide an environment in which healing can take place. In other words, ketones promote repair and reproduction of new brain cells.

Ketones have been shown to protect the brain from the formation of amyloid plaque deposits and cognitive decline seen in Alzheimer's disease in both animals and humans.[37-39] Ketones can act as histone deacetylase inhibitors—compounds that have long been used in psychiatry and neurology as mood stabilizers and antiepileptics, and more recently to treat cancer and inflammatory diseases.[40]

The ketogenic diet has received a good deal of attention as a harmless dietary treatment for cancer. The diet itself is said to starve cancer cells because cancer feeds on sugar (blood glucose). The ketogenic diet reduces blood sugar, switching the body's reliance from sugar to ketones. Cancer needs sugar to survive and cannot use ketones to produce energy; as a consequence, cancer cells essentially starve to death. This effect is caused by the dramatic reduction of carbohydrate in the diet and the body's shift to utilizing fat for its primary source of energy.

Ketones themselves can decrease tumor growth and viability even when blood glucose levels are high. So, their action on tumors is more involved than simply denying tumor cells sugar. In studies using mice with systemic metastatic cancer, ketone supplementation prolonged survival time independently of blood glucose levels or calorie consumption.[41] Part of the reason for this is that ketones themselves interfere with cancer cells' ability to absorb glucose and convert it to energy and help to restore apoptosis—programmed cell death—in cancer cells.[42] Ketones increase the sensitivity of cancer cells to radiation and chemotherapy and reduce the harmful side effects associated with these treatments.[43-44] This has led to the recommendation of using the ketogenic diet or ketone supplements in conjunction with standard cancer treatments as complementary therapies.

One of the most interesting characteristics of ketones is that they possess signaling activities, including the ability to affect gene expression; that is, they can make some genes more active and others less active. This is important because it can alter how cells respond to internal and environmental factors that affect health. Activation of certain genes can increase stress resistance and self-repair mechanisms, stimulate antioxidant production, and even extend lifespan.[45-47]

Ketones are produced whenever blood glucose levels decline. This occurs when food has not been eaten for awhile or when eating a very low-carbohydrate/ketogenic diet. Fasting and carbohydrate restriction can produce a moderate to high level of nutritional ketosis. Ketones are also produced during prolonged strenuous exercise as fat is utilized for energy. Exercise can raise blood ketones to mild levels. Consuming a source of medium chain triglycerides can also raise blood ketones to mild levels. The richest natural sources of MCTs are coconut and palm kernel oils. A product called MCT oil, derived from these oils, provides a higher concentration of MCTs. MCTs are metabolized differently from other fats, and in the process much of them are automatically converted into ketones by the liver, regardless of blood glucose levels. Consuming a source of MCTs can raise blood ketones even when a person is eating a typical high-carb diet. Adding coconut or MCT oil to a ketogenic diet can enhance ketone production.

Another way to raise blood ketones is with the use of exogenous ketone dietary supplements. Unlike MCTs, which are converted into ketones in our bodies, exogenous ketones need no conversion. They go directly into the bloodstream and can raise ketones to mild or moderate levels.

Ketone supplements, MCTs, and strenuous exercise produce short-term ketosis that only lasts a few hours at most. Fasting and eating a ketogenic diet produces a state of continual ketosis and remains as long as carbohydrate consumption is restricted. Some people combine all these methods to boost their ketone levels.

GOING KETO

The easiest way to get into ketosis using the ketogenic diet is to focus on carbohydrate restriction. Mild to moderate nutritional ketosis can usually be achieved by limiting total net carbohydrate intake to about 30 grams or less. Net carbohydrate means the carbohydrate that is absorbed and provides calories. Dietary fiber is also a carbohydrate, but it provides negligible calories. The nutrition facts label on foods lists total carbohydrate, which includes fiber. You can subtract the fiber grams from total carbohydrate grams to get net carbohydrate grams per serving. This is the number you use for calculating your total carbohydrate intake for the day.

Thirty grams is not much, so it is wise to eliminate all foods rich in starch and sugar. This includes all grains (wheat, rice, barley, corn, oats, etc.), potatoes, legumes, most fruits and all dried fruit, and all sweetened foods and beverages. The diet should be centered on low-carb or high-fiber vegetables, supplemented by meat, fish, eggs, cheese, and nuts, with some low-carb fruits. The foods are much the same as those eaten in a typical low-carb diet, but with some added refinements required to trigger the production of ketones.

Eating a big steak without any accompanying plant foods may be low-carb—actually, very low carb—but it is not ketogenic. Unlike many low-carb diets, the ketogenic diet is not a high-protein diet or a heavy meat diet. Protein intake is kept to modest levels at around 15 percent of total calorie intake. Physically active people can increase this to about 20 to 25 percent of calories. Normally, protein would be limited to about 60 to 90 grams per day. A lean 3 ounce (85 g) beefsteak, which is about the size of a deck of playing cards, supplies 21 grams of protein and a 3 ounce (85 g) chicken breast contains 26 grams of protein. The reason protein must be kept modest is that excess protein can be converted into glucose in the body. So, eating too much protein can have the same effect as eating carbohydrate. A high-protein diet will raise blood glucose levels and prevent the production of ketones.

Another distinction between the ketogenic diet and a low-carb diet is the addition of fat. Most low-carb diets are also moderately high in fat as well. This is because the meat and dairy that generally accompany a low-carb diet boost total fat intake. The ketogenic diet, however, purposely adds fats to raise total fat intake to 60 percent or more of calories. The fat is needed to supply energy due to the reduction in carbohydrate calories. Also, when in a state of ketosis, much of the fat in the diet is converted into ketones.

Fat is supplied by cooking and salad oils, animal fats, fatty meats, butter, full-fat dairy, cream, cheese, eggs, avocado, nuts, gravies and sauces, and other high-fat foods. Fats and oils should be used liberally in meal preparation. Eat the fat on meats and the skin on chicken. Don't be afraid of eating as much fat as you like.

Ketogenic diets used in the treatment of serious illnesses, such as epilepsy or cancer, require precise measurement of each macronutrient (carbohydrate, protein, and fat). If the macronutrients are not calculated for each meal, over time it is easy to slowly increase carbohydrate or protein intake and reduce fat intake, turning the ketogenic diet into an ordinary low-carb diet, which does not produce the ketones necessary to treat these conditions successfully.

A ketogenic diet used for weight loss, to improve blood glucose and insulin levels, treat minor health issues, and improve overall health, does not have to be as precise. As a general rule of thumb, for an average size adult with moderate activity level, a mild to moderate level of nutritional ketosis can be achieved and maintained by limiting total daily carbohydrate intake to 30 to 40 grams and protein to 60 to 90 grams, without limiting fat intake.

Many keto recipes in books and on the internet list the number of grams of carbohydrate, protein, and fat, as well as calories per serving. Packaged foods provide nutrition facts information on the container. If you make your own meals from fresh ingredients, you can use a table of nutrient values to calculate the net carbs and other nutrients. An easy-to-use, open-access nutrient chart listing fresh produce, grains, meat, and dairy can be accessed at www.coconutresearchcenter.org (look under the heading Ketogenic Diet). A good nutrient calculator with data on both fresh and processed foods can be accessed for free at www.calorieking.com. An excellent calculator available for a reasonable fee is www.carbmanager.com.

The ketogenic diet received its name from the fact that it produces ketones. If the diet does not produce ketones, it is not ketogenic. It takes about 3 to 6 days on the ketogenic diet before your ketone levels are elevated enough to measure at home. This is easily done with a urine ketosis test strip. The strips have one end that is chemically treated. When this end is dipped into a fresh specimen of urine it changes color depending on the ketone concentration in the urine. Using the test strip, you can tell if your blood ketone level is "none," "trace," "small," "moderate" or "large." The test is helpful in that it indicates if your diet is ketogenic and to what degree. You don't need to have a large level, small to moderate is adequate. These test strips are available at any pharmacy and are relatively inexpensive. There are other ketone testing devices that use blood samples or analyze the breath, and although they are more accurate, they are much more expensive and generally unnecessary.

If you plan on going on a ketogenic diet, it is highly advisable to use a testing device to make sure the diet actually gets you into nutritional ketosis. It is the only sure way to tell. Every person is a little different. Some people can get into a moderate level of ketosis by limiting carbohydrate intake to 40 grams a day, while another person may need to limit intake to 25 or 30 grams to achieve the same level of ketosis. So, you cannot judge yourself by the response of others. Ketosis test strips will be your guide.

When you go on a ketogenic diet, you need to stay on it for a designated period of time. In other words, you cannot cheat, as you might with a low-carb or low-fat diet. If you eat a piece of cake or some other high-carb food, it will throw you out of ketosis. Your ketosis test strips will indicate "zero," and you will need to spend another 2 to 3 days on the ketogenic diet before getting back into ketosis. Cheating just isn't worth it. Eating foods sweetened with zero-calorie sweeteners won't help you. They too can throw you out of ketosis or greatly reduce your ketone levels. All nonnutritive sweeteners are anti-ketogenic and will seriously affect your ketone levels.[48] The biggest mistake many people make when they go on a ketogenic diet is to think that because nonnutritive sweeteners are sugar- and calorie-free, they have no effect on blood sugar and insulin levels. Big mistake. Nonnutritive sweeteners can shut down ketone production in the liver and continue to affect ketone production until they are flushed out of the body.

The ketogenic diet does take effort to do properly, and if you are using the diet to treat a serious condition, it is necessary to make sure your diet is producing ketones. However, many people do not want to take the time or effort or worry about whether or not they are in ketosis. Yet they want to better manage their blood sugar and insulin levels and take advantage of having added fat in their diet. This way of eating is commonly referred to as a low-carb, high-fat (LCHF) diet. With the LCHF diet you are primarily concerned only about the amount of carbohydrate eaten, without worrying about protein intake. Such diets are generally high in meats, eggs, and dairy and consequently, also high in fat. Typically, high-fat foods are added to increase the total fat intake. LCHF diets that include a lot of protein do not produce ketones, and therefore, are not ketogenic.

You can continue all of your normal activities on the ketogenic diet. The first week you may experience a drop in your energy levels. This occurs as your body learns how to burn ketones and fatty acids as its primary source of fuel in place of glucose. Even on a low-carb diet the body burns glucose as its primary source of fuel. It takes about two weeks for the body to completely adapt to running on fat. Once that happens, your energy levels will rebound to pre-keto levels. You may actually experience increased energy and better endurance as your body burns fat instead of glucose. Many endurance athletes have discovered their performance times and endurance levels increase when eating a ketogenic diet.[49]

The ketogenic diet is generally considered to be a temporary therapeutic diet rather than a permanent eating plan. The ketogenic diet can be maintained long-term and even for a lifetime. For some serious conditions, such as epilepsy, patients remain on the diet for a couple of years, and in some cases, such as Alzheimer's or Parkinson's, patients may need to stay with it for life. However, for most circumstances the diet is best used for shorter periods of time and repeated periodically. This is referred to as keto cycling.

The therapeutic effects of the diet are more pronounced when you periodically cycle in and out of ketosis rather than remain in ketosis continually for long periods of time. Also, cycling allows you to plan when you will be in ketosis and when you are not. This way you can plan special events, such as birthdays and holidays, when you are out of ketosis so that you can enjoy the festivities without disrupting your diet. So, it is best to plan ahead when you know you would be likely to deviate from the diet.

The time spent in ketosis can vary from a few weeks to a few months, separated by a period of eating a normal, but healthy, diet. The ketogenic diet would be repeated as often as needed to achieve and maintain a person's health goals. You can learn more about the ketogenic diet and keto cycling in my book *Ketone Therapy: The Ketogenic Cleanse and Anti-Aging Diet.*

CONCLUSION

By now it should be clear that the overconsumption of sugar and refined starch are at the heart of our obesity epidemic and the underlying cause of metabolic syndrome and all of the chronic diseases associated with it. It should also be clear that for the most part fats are not the evil villains but essential nutrients that can promote better health, especially when they replace carbohydrate in the diet.

If you are currently eating a typical high-carb diet loaded with sugar and refined starch, you likely have some health concerns. If you are young and lucky enough not to be suffering from some type of chronic disease yet, it won't be long before you do.

The best thing you can do for your health is to eliminate or greatly reduce your sugar intake. Nonnutritive sweeteners should also be avoided completely. The biggest mistake many people make when they go on a low-carb diet is to substitute nonnutritive sweeteners for sugar. This doesn't help. Nonnutritive sweeteners keep sugar addiction alive and cause more harm than sugar does. Candy and sweets are the most obvious source of sugar and have no place in a healthy diet. For many people, the biggest source of sugar and nonnutritive sweeteners in their diet is beverages—soda, fruit-flavored drinks, sports drinks, and the like. Eliminating these would go a long way in reducing their sugar intake. Another major source of sugar is refined grain products—breakfast cereals, pastries, cookies, crackers, cakes, snack foods, and even breads. Get into the habit of reading ingredient labels. You would be surprised how much sugar is added to foods. Choose sugar-free options, without zero-calorie sweeteners. Reducing sugar, sweets, and refined grains from your diet is the most important step you can take toward a healthier diet.

You may be wondering: are there any sweeteners that are healthy, or perhaps benign, or at least less harmful? Unfortunately, no. There is no such thing as a "healthy" sweetener, and probably never will be. Some sweeteners may be a little better than others, but none could be termed healthy. Believe it or not, sugar, or at least some forms of it, is a better option than any of the low-calorie sugar substitutes.

Our bodies were programmed to associate the sweet taste with a corresponding amount of calories. Our bodies know how to process and utilize sugar to produce energy. In fact, every cell in your body knows how to metabolize sugar; it's the primary fuel that keeps us alive. Sugar is found in all plants. It is an essential component of mother's milk. It is a natural part of the human diet. That is more than you can say for any of the sugar substitutes. The primary problem with sugar is that we have discovered how to refine it, concentrate it, and use it to make treats and desserts. Sugary foods are around us everywhere. It is far too easy to become addicted to sugar, and many of us are. It is the addiction, and overconsumption, that makes sugar so detrimental.

As noted earlier, on average we each consume about 130 pounds (59 kg) of added sugar a year. That amounts to about 40 teaspoons of sugar a day! No wonder sugar is associated with so many health problems. Anything consumed in huge amounts can be harmful.

The US Department of Agriculture (USDA) recommends that we limit our added sugar intake to no more than 6 percent of total calories consumed. For a typical 2,000 calorie diet, that would equate to 32 grams, or 8 teaspoons of sugar per day.[50] The American Heart Association recommends that men limit their added sugar intake to 9 teaspoons or less, which is equivalent to 36 grams or 150 calories; and women limit their intake to 6 teaspoons or less, which is equivalent to 25 grams or 100 calories.[51] These quantities would be far below the average, and sensible limits for most people. If you have diabetes, it would be wise to eliminate all sugar from your diet, including the sugar that is added to processed foods, so you would need to read the Nutrition Facts panel on the package to know how much sugar there is in each serving. Unprocessed fresh foods don't have any added sugar. By eliminating nonnutritive sweeteners and reducing the amount of sugar you eat, you will also limit your consumption of processed, poor-quality foods, which will help tremendously in your quest for better health.

If you eat a little sugar, the type of sugar you eat is also important. Natural or minimally processed sugars are preferred over highly processed ones. Fructose is one of the most highly processed, and is absolutely the worst in terms of what it does to your health. Fructose is just as bad for you as any of the noncaloric sweeteners. Avoid all high fructose sweeteners, including corn syrup, high-fructose corn syrup, and agave.

Natural sweeteners are somewhat better than refined sugar because they contain a small quantity of vitamins and minerals, so they are not completely empty calories. The best natural sweeteners include maple sugar/syrup, coconut sugar/syrup, raw honey, dehydrated sugarcane juice (Sucanat, rapadura, panela, jaggery, and muscovado), date sugar, brown rice syrup, and barley malt syrup. If you must use something to sweeten your food, your best choice would be one of these natural sweeteners, and to limit it to 8 or less teaspoons a day.

The next step you can take to improve your health is to go on a low-carb diet by restricting total carbohydrate consumption to fewer than 150 or 100 grams per day. This would require reducing or eliminating additional foods, such as sweetened dairy (yogurt, chocolate milk, ice cream, etc.) and all grains and bread products. Starchy vegetables such as potatoes and legumes would also need to be restricted.

Don't be afraid to add more fat into your diet. Choose full-fat foods, whole milk, cheese, and cream. Add fats liberally to your foods. Use butter liberally, and add bacon drippings and other fats to your cooking. Your meals will taste much better. Use saturated and monounsaturated fats in your cooking. Avoid polyunsaturated vegetable oils, as they degrade too quickly in cooking and form unhealthy by-products. Add some fish, shellfish, seaweed, leafy greens, free-range eggs, and organic grass-fed meats to your weekly diet to get your omega-3 fatty acids. Avoid all products containing hydrogenated vegetable oil. Read ingredient labels.

Replace the sugar and grains you remove from your diet with more non-starchy vegetables of all types. Most people tend to shy away from vegetables because they grew up eating them boiled or cooked in a steamer, seasoned only with salt and a few seasonings. Butter and other fats were out because they were perceived as unhealthy. Consequently, the vegetables were generally bland and unappetizing. Vegetables can be delicious. Use butter, bacon drippings, and other fats, as well as gravies and sauces to enhance the natural flavor of the vegetables. It is amazing how appetizing vegetables can taste when prepared properly. A good source of low-carb/ketogenic vegetable recipes is my book *Dr. Fife's Keto Cookery*. The book contains 450 ketogenic recipes, including 70 vegetable recipes and 50 delicious high-fat sauces. Each recipe includes the nutrient content so you know exactly how much carbohydrate, protein, and fat is in each serving.

If you suffer from degenerative or chronic health problems or take medications for high blood pressure, diabetes, high cholesterol, and such, you should consider going to the next step—a ketogenic diet—and reduce your carbohydrate intake to about 30 grams per day. You will experience some incredible improvements and likely be able to greatly reduce or even eliminate your medications.

For additional information about the ketogenic diet and the health and nutritional aspects of fats and oils, visit my website Coconut Research Center at www.coconutresearchcenter.org.

References

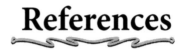

Chapter 1: A Big Fat Mistake
1. http://www.alz.org/facts/

Chapter 2: Modern Diets and Degenerative Disease
1. Gutteridge, RP and Halliwell, B. *Antioxidants in Nutrition, Health, and Disease.* Oxford University Press: Oxford; 1994.
2. Brennan, RO. *Nutrigenetics.* New York: Evans and Co, Inc. 1975.
3. McGee, CT. *Heart Frauds: Uncovering the Biggest Health Scam in History.* Piccadilly Books, Ltd: Colorado Springs, Colorado; 2007.
4. Price, WA. *Nutrition and Physical Degeneration*, New Cannan, CT: Keats Pub 1945.
5. Prior, IAM. The price of civilization. *Nutrition Today* July/Aug;1971:2-11.
6. Schaefer, O. When the Eskimo Comes to Town. *Nutrition Today*.1971;6:8-16.
7. Malhotra, A, et al. It is time to bust the myth of physical inactivity and obesity: you cannot outrun a bad diet. *British J Sports Med* 2015:49:967-968.

Chapter 3: The War On Fat
1. White, PD. *Prog Cardiovascular Dis* 1971;14:249.
2. Keys, A. Atherosclerosis: A problem in newer public health. *Journal of Mount Sinai Hospital* 1953;20:118-139.
3. Yerushalmy, J and Hilleboe, HE. Fat in the diet and mortality from heart disease. A methodologic note. *The New York State Journal of Medicine* 1957;2343-2354.
4. Yudkin, J. *Sweet and Dangerous.* Bantam: New York, 1972.
5. Yudkin, J. Sucrose and heart disease. *Nutrition Today* Spring;1969:16-20.
6. Leren, P. The effect of a cholesterol lowering diet in male survivors of myocardial infarction. (A controlled clinical trial). *Nord Med* 1967;25;77:658-661.
7. Yudkin, J and Roddy, J. Levels of dietary sucrose in patients with occlusive atherosclerotic disease. *Lancet* 1964;2:6-8.
8. Yudkin, J. Diet and coronary thrombosis hypothesis and fact. *Lancet* 1957;273:155-162.
9. Cohen, AM. Fats and carbohydrates as factors in atherosclerosis and diabetes in Yemenite Jews. *Am Heart J* 1963;65:291-293.
10. Armstrong, BK, et al. Commodity consumption and ischemic heart disease mortality, with special reference to dietary practices. *J Chron Dis* 1975;28:455-469.
11. Page IH, et al. Dietary fat and its relation to heart attacks and strokes. Report by the Central Committee for Medical and Community Program of the American Heart Association. *Circulation* 1961;23:133-136.
12. Keys, A. The age trend of serum concentrations of cholesterol and of Sf 10-20 ("G") substances in Adults. *J Gerontol* 1952;7: 201-206.

13. Frantz, ID, JR, et al. Test of effect of lipid lowering by diet on cardiovascular risk. The Minnesota Coronary Survey. 1989. *Arteriosclerosis* 9:129-135.

14. Ramsden, CE, et al. Re-evaluation of the traditional diet-heart hypothesis: analysis of recovered data for Minnesota Coronary Experiment (1968-73). *BMJ* 2016;353:i1246.

15. http://www.motherjones.com/environment/2012/10/former-dentist-sugar-industry-lies. Kearns, CK. How a former dentist drilled the sugar industry. *Mother Jones* Oct 13, 2012.

16. O'Neil, C, et al. Association of candy consumption with body weight measures, other health risk factors for cardiovascular disease, and diet quality in US children and adolescents: NHANES 1999-2004. *Food & Nutrition Research* 2011;55. doi: 10.3402/fnr.v55i0.5794.

Chapter 4: Sugar Isn't Always Sweet

1. Whitney, EN, et al. *Understanding Normal and Clinical Nutrition, Third Edition.* West Publishing Company, St. Paul, MN, 1991.

2. Warram, JH, et al. Slow glucose removal rate and hyperinsulinemia precede the development of type 2 diabetes in the offspring of diabetic parents. *Ann Intern Med* 1990;113:909-915.

3. Malik, VS, et al. Sugar-sweetened beverages and risk of metabolic syndrome and type 2 diabetes. *Diabetes Care* 2010; 33(11): 2477-2483.

4. Basu, S, et al. The relationship of sugar to population-level diabetes prevalence: an econometric analysis of repeated cross-sectional data. *PLoS One* 2013;8:e57873.

5. Liu, S, et al. Relation between a diet with a high glycemic load and plasma concentrations of high-sensitivity C-reactive protein in middle-aged women. *Am J Clin Nutr* 2002;75:492-498.

6. Dickinson, S, et al. High glycemic index carbohydrate mediates an acute proinflammatory process as measured by NF-kappaB activation. *Asia Pac J Clin Nutr* 2005;14Suppl:S120.

7. Ridker, P, et al. C-reactive protein and other markers of inflammation in the prediction of cardiovascular disease in women. *N Engl J Med* 2000;342(12):836-843.

8. Sasaki, N, et al. Advanced glycation end products in Alzheimer's disease and other neurodegenerative diseases. *American Journal of Pathology* 1998;153:1149-1155.

9. Catellani, R, et al. Glycooxidation and oxidative stress in Parkinson's disease and diffuse Lewy body disease. *Brain Res* 1996;737:195-200.

10. Kato, S, et al. Astrocytic hyaline inclusions contain advanced glycation end-products in familial amyotrophic lateral sclerosis with superoxide dismutase 1 gene mutation: immunohistochemical and immunoelectron microscopical analysis. *Aca Neuropathol* 1999;97:260-266.

11. The Diabetes Control and Complications Trial Research Group. The effect of intensive treatment of diabetes on the development and progression of long-term complications in insulin-dependent diabetes mellitus. *N Engl J Med* 1993;329:977-986.

12. Haffner, SM, et al. Mortality from coronary heart disease in subjects with type 2 diabetes and in nondiabetic subjects with and without prior myocardial infarction. *N Engl J Med* 1998;339:229-234.

13. Turner, RC, et al. Risk factors for coronary artery disease in non-insulin dependent diabetes mellitus: United Kingdom Prospective Diabetes Study (UKPDS: 23) *BMJ* 1998;316:823-828.

14. De Vegt, F, et al. Hyperglycaemia is associated with all-cause and cardiovascular mortality in the Hoorn population: the Hoorn Study. *Diabetologia* 1999;42:926-931.

15. Basta, G, et al. Advanced glycation end products and vascular inflammation: implications for accelerated atherosclerosis in diabetes. *Cardiovascular Research* 2004;63:582-592.

16. Kanauchi, M, et al. Advanced glycation end products in nondiabetic patients with coronary artery disease. *Diabetes Care* 2001;24:1620-1623.

17. Kiuchi, K, et al. Increased serum concentrations of advanced glycation end products: a marker of coronary artery disease activity in type 2 diabetic patients. *Heart* 2001;85:87-91.

18. Won, KB, et al. High serum advanced glycation end-products predict coronary artery disease irrespective of arterial stiffness in diabetic patients. *Korean Circ J* 2012;42:335-340.

19. Stirban, A, et al. Vascular effects of advanced glycation endproducts: clinical effects and molecular mechanisms. *Molecular Metabolism* 2014;3:94-108.

20. Goldberg, T, et al. Advanced glycoxidation end products in commonly consumed foods. *J Am Diet Assoc* 2004;104:1287-1291.

21. Uribarri, J, et al. Circulating glycotoxins and dietary advanced glycation endproducts: two links to inflammatory response, oxidative stress, and aging. *J Gerontol Ser A: Biol Sci Med Sci* 2007;62:427-433.

22. Krajcovicová-Kudlacková, M., et al. Advanced glycation end products and nutrition. *Physiol Res* 2002;51:313-316.

23. Forristal, LJ. 2001. The murky world of high fructose corn syrup. *Wise Traditions* 2(3):60-61.

24. Ouyang, X, et al. Fructose consumption as a risk factor for non-alcoholic fatty liver disease. *J Hepatol* 2008;48:993-999.

25. Abdelmalek, MF, et al. Increased fructose consumption is associated with fibrosis severity in patients with nonalcoholic fatty liver disease. *Hepatology* 2010;51:1961-1971.

26. Bocarsly, M.E., et al. High-fructose corn syrup causes characteristics of obesity in rats: increased body weight, body fat and triglyceride levels. *Pharmacol Biochem Behav* 2010;97:101-106.

27. Princeton University, "High-Fructose Corn Syrup Prompts Considerably More Weight Gain, Researchers Find," *Science Daily*, March 22, 2010.

28. Reiser, S, et al. 1985. Indices of copper status in humans consuming a typical American diet containing either fructose or starch. *Am J Clin Nutr* 42(2):242-251.

29. http://www.thinkusadairy.org/products/milk-powders/milk-powder-categories/non-fat-dry-milk-and-skim-milk-powder.

30. Bo-Htay, C, et al. Effects of D-galactose-induced ageing on the heart and its potential interventions. *J Cell Mol Med* 2018;22:1392-1410.

31. Armstrong, BK, et al. Commodity consumption and ischemic heart disease mortality, with special reference to dietary practices. *J Chron Dis* 1975;28:455-469.

32. Grant, WB. Milk and other dietary influences on coronary heart disease. *Altern Med Rev* 1998;3:281-294.

33. Michaelsson, K, et al. Milk intake and risk of mortality and fractures in women and men: cohort studies. *BMJ* 2014;349.g6015.

34. Fox, PF and McSweeney, P. *Advanced Dairy Chemisty: Volume 2, Lipids,* Birkhauser; 2006:655.

35. Hubbard, RW, et al. Atherogenic effect of oxidized products of cholesterol. *Progress in Food & Nutrition Science* 1989;13:17-44.

Chapter 5: A Weapon of Mass Destruction

1. World Health Organization, "Noncommunicable Diseases," fact sheet, World Health Organization website, June 1, 2018, http://www.who.int/news-room/fact-sheets/detail/noncommunicable-diseases.

2. Magalle, L, et al. Intense sweetness surpasses cocaine reward. *PLoS One* 2007;8:e698.

3. Gearhardt, AN, et al. Neural correlates of food addiction. *Arch Gen Psychiatry* 2011;68:808-816.

4. http://bmjopen.bmj.com/content/6/3/e009892.

5. Martinez Steele, E, et al. Ultra-processed foods and added sugars in the US diet: evidence from a nationally representative cross-section al study. *BMJ Open* 2016 Mar 9;6(3):e009892. doi: 10.1136/bmjopen-2015-009892.

6. Cheraskin, E, et al. Effect of low-refined-carbohydrate diet upon vitamin C state. *Internat J Vit Res* 1970;40:77-80.

7. Verhoef, P, et al. Plasma total homocysteine, B vitamins, and risk of coronary atherosclerosis. *Arteriosclerosis, Thrombosis, and Vascular Biology* 1997;17:989-995.

8. Kekwick, A and Pawan, GLS. Calorie intake in relation to body weight changes in the obese. Lancet 1956;1:155.

9. Hu, F.B. and Malik, V.S. Sugar-sweetened beverages and risk of obesity and type 2 diabetes: epidemiologic evidence. *Physiol Behav* 2010;100:47-54.

10. Stranahan, AM, et al. Diet-induced insulin resistance impairs hippocampal synaptic plasticity and cognition in middle-aged rats. *Hippocampus* 2008;18:1085-1088.

11. Cao, D, et al. Intake of sucrose-sweetened water induces insulin resistance and exacerbates memory deficits and amyloidosis in a transgenic mouse model of Alzheimer disease. *J Biol Chem* 2007;282:36275-36282.

12. Xu, W, et al. Mid- and late-life diabetes in relation to the risk of dementia: a population-based twin study. *Diabetes* 2009;58:71-77.

13. Pavlovic, DM and Pavlovic, AM. Dementia and diabetes mellitus. *Srp Arh Celok Lek* 2008;136:170-175.

14. Ristow, M. Neurodegenerative disorders associated with diabetes mellitus. *J Mol Med* 2004;82:510-529.

15. Craft, S and Watson, G.S. Insulin and neurodegenerative disease: shared and specific mechanisms. *Lancet Neurol* 2004;3:169-178.

16. Reyes, ET, et al Insulin resistance in amyotrophic lateral sclerosis. *J Neurol Sci* 1984;63:317-324.

17. Hu, G, et al. Type 2 diabetes and the risk of Parkinson's disease. *Diabetes Care* 2007;30:842-847.

18. Sandyk, R. The relationship between diabetes mellitus and Parkinson's disease. *Int. J Neurosci* 1993;69:125-130.

19. Moroo, I, et al. Loss of insulin receptor immunoreactivity from the substantia nigra pars compacta neurons in Parkinson's disease. *Acta Neuropathol* 1994;87:343-348.

20. Sandyk, R. The relationship between diabetes mellitus and Parkinson's disease. *Int J Neurosci* 1993;69:125-130.

21. Hubbard, RW, et al. Elevated plasma glucagon in amyotrophic lateral sclerosis. *Neurology* 1992;42:1532-1534.

22. Farrer, L.A. Diabetes mellitus in Huntington's disease. *Clin Genet* 1985;27:62-67.

23. Podolsky, S, et al. Increased frequency of diabetes mellitus in patients with Huntington's chorea. *Lancet* 1972;1:1356-1358.

24. Rodriguez, RR and Krehal, WA. The influence of diet and insulin on the incidence of cataracts in diabetic rats. *Yale J Biol Med* 1951;24:103-108.

25. The effect of intensive treatment of diabetes on the development and progression of long-term complications in insulin-dependent diabetes mellitus. The Diabetes Control and Complications Research Group. *N Engl J Med* 1993;329:977-986.

26. Chiu, CJ, et al. Carbohydrate intake and glycemic index in relation to the odds of early cortical and nuclear lens opacities. *Am J Clin Nutr* 2005;81:1411-1416.

27. Stratton, IM, et al. Association of glycaemia with macrovascular and microvascular complications of type 2 diabetes (UKPDS 35): prospective observational study. *BMJ* 2000;321:405-412.

28. The effect of intensive diabetes treatment on the progression of diabetic retinopathy in insulin-dependent diabetes mellitus. The Diabetes Control and Complications Trial. *Arch Ophthalmol* 1995;113:36-51.

29. Kerti, L, et al. Higher glucose levels associated with lower memory and reduced hippocampal microstructure. *Neurology* 2013;81:1745-1752.

30. Warram, JH, et al. Slow glucose removal rate and hyperinsulinemia precede the development of type 2 diabetes in the offspring of diabetic parents. *Ann Intern Med* 1990;113:909-915.

31. Hamer, HM, et al. Review article: the role of butyrate on colonic function. *Aliment Pharmacol Ther* 2008;27:104-119.

32. Hu, GX, et al. Activation of the AMP activated protein kinase by short-chain fatty acids is the main mechanism underlying the beneficial effect of a high fiber diet on the metabolic syndrome. *Med Hypotheses* 2010;74:123-126.

33. Gao, Z, et al. Butyrate improves insulin sensitivity and increases energy expenditure in mice. *Diabetes* 2009;58:1509-1517.

34. Blouin, JM, et al. Butyrate elicits a metabolic switch in human colon cancer cells by targeting the pyruvate dehydrogenase complex. *Int J Cancer* 2001;128:2591-2601.

35. Harig, J M, et al. Treatment of diversion colitis with short-chain-fatty acid irrigation. *N Engl J Med* 1989;320: 23-28.

36. Di Sabatino, A, et al. Oral butyrate for mildly to moderately active Crohn's disease. *Alimen. Pharmacol Ther* 2005;22: 789-794.

37. Binder, H J. Role of colonic short-chain fatty acid transport in diarrhea. *Annu Rev Physiol* 2010:72: 297-313.

38. Pihlstrom, BL, et al. Periodontal diseases. *Lancet* 2005;366:1809-1820.

39. Kirdis, E, et al. Ribonucleotide reductase class III, an essential enzyme for the anaerobic growth of Staphylococcus aureus, is a virulence determinant in septic arthritis. *Microb Pathog* 2007:43:179-188.

40. Rams, TE and Slots, J. Systemic manifestations of oral infections. In: *Contemporary Oral Microbiology and Immunology*. Slots J., Taubaman, M.A. editors. St. Louis: Mosby, 1992;500-510.

41. Van Dyke, TE, et al. Potential role of microorganisms isolated from periodontal lesions in the pathogenesis of inflammatory bowel disease. *Infect Immun* 1986;53:671-677.

42. Lerner, UH. Inflammation-induced bone remodeling in periodontal disease and the influence of post-menopausal osteoporosis. *J Dent Res* 2006;85:596-607.

43. Mealey, B.L. and Rethman, M.P. Periodontal disease and diabetes mellitus. Bidirectional relationship. *Dent Today* 2003;22:107-113.

44. Lacopino, AM. Periodontitis and diabetes interrelationships: role of inflammation. *Ann Periodontol* 2001;6:125-137.

45. Offenbacher, S, et al. Periodontal infection as a risk factor for preterm low birth weight. *J Periodont* 1996;67(10 Suppl):1103-1113.

46. Kozarov, EV, et al. Human atherosclerotic plaque contains viable invasive Actinobacillus actinomycetemcomitans and Porphyromonas gingivalis. *Arterioscler Thromb Vasc Biol* 2005;25:17-18.

47.Mattila, KJ, et al. Dental infections and cardiovascular diseases: a review. *J Periodontol* 2005;76(11Suppl):2085-2088.

48. Anonymous. Bad teeth and gums a risk factor for heart disease? *Harvard Heart Letter* 1998;9:6.

49. Millman, C. The route of all evil. *Men's Health* 1999;14:102.

50. DeStefano, F, et al. Dental disease and risk of coronary heart disease and mortality. *BMJ* 1993;306:688-691.

51. Morrison, HI, et al. Periodontal disease and risk of fatal coronary heart and cerebrovascular diseases. *J Cardiovasc Risk* 1999;6:7-11.

52. Loesche, W, et al. Assessing the relationship between dental disease and coronary heart disease in elderly U.S. veterans. *J Am Dent Assoc* 1998;129:301-311.

53. Pucher, J and Stewart, J. Periodontal disease and diabetes mellitus. *Curr Diab Rep* 2004;4:46-50.

54. Iacopino, AM. Periodontitis and diabetes interrelationships: role of inflammation. *Ann Periodontol* 2001;6:125-137.

55. Mealey, BL and Rose, LF. Diabetes mellitus and inflammatory periodontal diseases. *Curr Opin Endocrinol Diabetes Obes* 2008;15:135-141.

56.Satish BN, Srikala P, Maharudrappa B et al. Saliva: a tool in assessing glucose levels in diabetes mellitus. *J Int Oral Health* 2014; 6 (2): 114–117.

57. Noble, JM, et al. Periodontitis is associated with cognitive impairment among older adults: analysis of NHANES-III. *J Neurol Neurosurg Psychiatry* 2009;80:1206-1211.

58. Ellefsen, B, et al. Caries prevalence in older persons with and without dementia. *J Am Geriatr Soc* 2008;56:59-67.

59.Hanaoka, A. and Kashihara, K. Increased frequencies of caries, periodontal disease and tooth loss in patients with Parkinson's disease. *Journal of Clinical Neuroscience* 2009;16:1279-1282.

60. Galata, G. Results in a case of Parkinson's disease due to alveolar pyorrhea, treated with bismuth by parenteral route. *Policlinico Prat* 1964;71:220-223.

61. Stein, PS, et al. Tooth loss, dementia and neuropathology in the Nun Study. *J Am Dent Assoc* 2007;138:1314-1322.

62. Gatz, M, et al. Potentially modifiable risk factors for dementia in identical twins. *Alzheimer Dement* 2006;2:110-117.

63. Sanchez, A, et al. Role of sugars in human neutrophilic phagocytosis. *Am J Clin Nutr* 1973;26:1180-1184.

64. Holleb, A.I. *The American Cancer Society Cancer Book*. Doubleday & Company: New York, 1986.

65. Bertrand, KA, et al. Periodontal disease and risk of non-Hodgkin lymphoma in the health professionals follow-up study. *Int J Cancer* 2016;doi:10.1002/ijc.30518.

66. Yamamura, K, et al. human Microbiome Fusobacterium Nucleatum in esophageal cancer tissue is associated with prognosis. *Clin Cancer Res* 2016, Oct 21.

67. Fan, X, et al. Human oral microbiome and prospective risk for pancreatic cancer: a population-based nested case-control study. *Gut* 2016, Oct 14.

68. Momen-Heravi, F, et al. Periodontal disease, tooth loss and colorectal cancer risk: results from the Nurses' Health Study. *Int J Cancer* 2016, Oct 25.

69. Zeng, XT, et al. Periodontal disease and incident lung cancer risk: a meta-analysis of cohort studies. *J Periodontol* 2016;87:1158-1164.

70. Michaud, DS, et al. Periodontal disease, tooth loss, and cancer risk in a prospective study of male health professionals. *Lancet Oncol* 2008;9:550-558.

71. Higginbotham, S., et al. Dietary glycemic load and risk of colorectal cancer in the Women's Health Study. *Journal of the National Cancer Institute* 2004;96:229-233.

72. Smith, U and Gale, EM. Cancer and diabetes: are we ready for prime time? *Diabetologia* 2010;53:1541-1544.

73. https://www.cancer.org/cancer/non-small-cell-lung-cancer/about/key-statistics.html.

74. https://www.lung.org/lung-health-and-diseases/lung-disease-lookup/lung-cancer/resource-library/lung-cancer-fact-sheet.html.

75. Stefansson, V. *Cancer: Disease of Civilization?* Hill and Wang: New York, 1960.

76.Schaefer, O. Medical observations and problems in the Canadian arctic. *Canad M A J* 1959;81:386-393.

77. Fife, B. *Ketone Therapy: The Ketogenic Cleanse and Anti-Aging Diet*. Piccadilly Books, Ltd.: Colorado Springs, CO;2017.

78. Rapp, K, et al. Obestiy and incidence of cancer: a large cohort study of over 145,000 adults in Austria. *Br J Cancer* 2005;93:1062-1067.

79. Stocks, T, et al. Blood glucose and risk of incident and fatal cancer in the Metabolic Syndrome and Cancer Project (Me-Can): analysis of six prospective cohorts. *PLoS Med* 2009;6:e1000201.

80. Rapp, K, et al. Fasting blood glucose and cancer risk in a cohort of more than 140,000 adults in Austria. *Diabetologia* 2006;49:945-952.

Chapter 6: Metabolic Syndrome

1. Feinman, RD, et al. Dietary carbohydrate restriction as the first approach in diabetes management: Critical review and evidence base. *Nutrition* 2015;31:1-13.

2. Reaven, G. The metabolic syndrome or the insulin resistance syndrome? Different names, different concepts, and different goals. *Endocrinol Metab Clin North Am* 2004; 33: 283–303.

3. Larsson, B, et al. Abdominal adipose tissue distribution, obesity, and risk of cardiovascular disease and death: 13 year follow up of participants in the study of men born in 1913. *Br Med J (Clin Res Ed)* 1984;288:1401-1404.

4. Zhang, C, et al. Abdominal obesity and the risk of all-cause, cardiovascular, and cancer mortality: sixteen years of follow-up in US women. *Circulation* 2008;117:1658-67.

5. Ford, ES, et al. Prevalence of the metabolic syndrome among US adults: findings from the Third National Health and Nutrition Examination Survey. *JAMA* 2002; 287: 356–359.

6. Despres JP. Health consequences of visceral obesity. *Ann Med* 2001;33:534-41.

7. Hanley AJ, et al. Metabolic and inflammation variable clusters and prediction of type 2 diabetes: factor analysis using directly measured insulin sensitivity. *Diabetes* 2004; 53: 1773-1781.

8. Shulman, GI. Cellular mechanisms of insulin resistance. *J Clin Invest* 2000; 106: 171-176.

9. Hotamisligil, GS. Inflammatory pathways and insulin action. *Int J Obes Relat Metab Disord* 2003; 27 (suppl 3): S53-S55.

10. Ruan, H and Lodish, HF. Insulin resistance in adipose tissue: direct and indirect effects of tumor necrosis factor-alpha. *Cytokine Growth Factor Rev* 2003; 14: 447-455.

11. Welsh, JA, et al. Caloric sweetener consumption and dyslipidemia among US adults. *JAMA* 2010;303:1490-1497.

12. Stanhope, KL, et al. Consumption of fructose and high fructose corn syrup increase postprandial triglycerides, LDL-cholesterol, and apolipoprotein-B in young men and women. *J Clin Endocrinol Metab* 2011;96:E1596-E1605.

13. Xi, B, et al. Sugar-sweetened beverages and risk of hypertension and CVD: a dose-response meta-analysis. *Br J Nutr* 2015;113:709-717.

14. Lavi, T, et al. The acute effect of various glycemic index dietary carbohydrates on endothelial function in nondiabetic overweight and obese subjects. *J Am Coll Cardiol* 2009;53:2283-2287.

15. Chowdhury, R. et al. Association of dietary, circulating, and supplement fatty acids with coronary risk: a systematic review and meta-analysis. *Ann Intern Med* 2014;160:398-406.

16. Fan, J, et al. Dietary glycemic index, glycemic load, and risk of coronary heart disease, stroke, and stroke mortality: a systematic review with meta-analysis. *PLoS One* 2012;7:e52182.

17. Dehghan, M, et al. Associations of fats and carbohydrate intake with cardiovascular disease and mortality in 18 countries from five continents (PURE): a prospective cohort study. *Lancet* 2017;390:2050-2062.

18. Zarychanski, R, et al. Nonnutritive sweeteners and cardiometabolic health: a systematic review and meta-analysis of randomized controlled trials and prospective cohort studies. *CMAJ* 2017;189:E929-939.

19. Gardner C, et al. American Heart Association Nutrition Committee of the Council on Nutrition, Physical Activity and Metabolism, Council on Arteriosclerosis, Thrombosis and Vascular Biology, Council on Cardiovascular Disease in the Young; American Diabetes Association. Nonnutritive sweeteners: current use and health perspectives: a scientific statement from the American Heart Association and the American Diabetes Association. *Diabetes Care* 2012;35(8):1798-1808.

20. Swithers, SE. Artificial sweeteners produce the counterintuitive effect of inducing metabolic derangements. *Trends Endocrinol Metab* 2013;24:431-41.

21. Nettleton, JE, et al. Reshaping the gut microbiota: Impact of low calorie sweeteners and the link to insulin resistance? *Physiol Behav* 2016; 164(Pt B):488-93.

22. Fowler, SP. Low-calorie sweetener use and energy balance: results from experimental studies in animals, and large-scale prospective studies in humans. *Physiol Behav* 2016;164(Pt B):517-23.

23. Wang, Qiao-Ping, et al. Sucralose promotes food intake through NPY and a neuronal fasting response. *Cell Metabolism* 2016;24:75-90.

24. Bleich, SN, et al. Diet-beverage consumption and caloric intake among US adults, overall and by body weight. *Am J Public Health* 2014;104(3):e72-8.

25. Fife, B. *The Stevia Deception: The Hidden Dangers of Low-Calorie Sweeteners.* Piccadilly Books, Ltd.: Colorado Springs, CO., 2017.

26. Pase, MP, et al. Sugar- and artificially sweetened beverages and the risks of incident stroke and dementia. *Stroke* 2017;48:1139-1140.

27. https://now.uiowa.edu/2014/03/ui-study-finds-diet-drinks-associated-heart-trouble-older-women.

28. Proceedings of the European Association for the Study of Diabeetews, Lisbon, Portugal, September 13, 2017.

29. Suez, J, et al. Artificial sweeteners induce glucose intolerance by altering the gut microbiota. *Nature* 2014;514:181-186.

30. Harpar, D, et al. Measuring artificial sweeteners toxicity using a bioluminescent bacterial panel. *Molecules* 2018;23:2454.

31. Suez, J, et al. Artificial sweeteners induce glucose intolerance by altering the gut microbiota. *Nature* 2014;514:181-186.

32. Azad, Meghan B, et al. Association between artificially sweetened beverage consumption during pregnancy and infant body mass index. *JAMA Pediatrics* 2016;170:662-670.

Chapter 7: Understanding Fats

1. Samieri, C, et al. Low plasma eicosapentaenoic acid and depressive symptomatology are independent predictors of dementia risk. *Am J Clin Nutr* 2008;88:714-721.

2. Hibbeln, JR. Depression, suicide and deficiencies of omega-3 essential fatty acids in modern diets. *World Rev Nutr Diet* 2009;99:17-30.

3. Plourde, M and Cunnane, SC. Extremely limited synthesis of long chain polyunsaturates in adults: implications for their dietary essentiality and use as supplements. *Appl Physiol Nutr Metab* 2007;32:619-634.

4. Brunner, J, et al. Cholesterol, omega-3 fatty acids, and suicide risk: empirical evidence and pathophysiological hypotheses. *Fortschr Neurol Psychiatr* 2001;69:460-467.

5. Colin, A, et al. Lipids, depression and suicide. *Encephale* 2003;29:49-58.

6. Wells, AS, et al. Alterations in mood after changing to a low-fat diet. *Br J Nutr* 1998;79:23-30.

7. http://en.wikipedia.org/wiki;Life_expectancy.

8. McGee, D, et al. The relationship of dietary fat and cholesterol to mortality in 10 years: the Honolulu Heart Program. *Int J Epidemiol* 1985;14:97-105.

9. Okamoto, K., et al. Nutritional status and risk of amyotrophic lateral sclerosis in Japan. *Amyotroph Lateral Scler* 2007;8:300-304.

10. Forsythe, CE, et al. Comparison of low fat and low carbohydrate diets on circulating fatty acid composition and markers of inflammation. *Lipids* 2008;43:65-77.

11. de Souza, RJ, et al. Intake of saturated and trans unsaturated fatty acids and risk of all cause mortality, cardiovascular disease, and type 2 diabetes: systematic review and meta-analysis of observational studies. *BMJ* 2015;351:h3978.

12. https://www.issfal.org/assets/issfal%2003%20pufaintakereccomdfinalreport.pdf.

13. Barnard, ND. Trends in food availability, 1909–2007. *Am J Clin Nutr* 2010;91:1530S–1536S. doi: 10.3945/ajcn.2010.28701G.

14. Vangaveti, VN, et al. Hydroxyoctadecadienoic acids: Oxidised derivatives of linoleic acid and their role in inflammation associated with metabolic syndrome and cancer. *Eur J Pharmacol* 2016;785:70-76.

15. Ohmon, H, et al. Dietary linoleic acid and glucose enhances azoxymethane-induced colon cancer and metastases via the expression of high-mobility group box 1. *Pathobiology* 2010;77:210-217.

16. Ip, C, et al. Requirement of essential fatty acid for mammary tumorigenesis in the rat. *Cancer Res* 1985;45:1997-2001.

17. Liou, YA, et al. Decreasing linoleic acid with constant alpha-linolenic acid in dietary fats increases (n-3) eicosapentaenoic acid in plasma phospholipids in healthy men. *J Nutr* 2007;137:945-952.

18. Blasbalg, TL, et al. Changes in consumption of omega-3 and omega-6 fatty acids in the United States during the 20th century. *Am J Clin Nutr* 2011;93:950-962.

19. Keys, A, et al. Prediction of serum-cholesterol responses of man to changes in fats in the diet. *Lancet* 1957;273:959-966.

20. Chowdhury, R, et al. Association of dietary, circulating, and supplement fatty acids with coronary risk: a systematic review and meta-analysis. *Ann Intern Med* 2014;160:398-406.

21. Ramsden, DE, et al. Use of dietary linoleic acid for secondary prevention of coronary heart disease and death: Evaluation of recovered data from the Sydney Diet Heart Study and updated meta-analysis. *BMJ* 2013;346 doi:1136/bmj.e8707.
22. Blasbalg, TL, et al. Changes in consumption of omega-3 and omega-6 fatty acids in the United States during the 20th century. *Am J Clin Nutr* 2011;93:950-962.
23. Pamplona, R, et al. Low fatty acid unsaturation: a mechanism for lowered lipoperoxidative modification of tissue proteins in mammalian species with long life spans. *J Gerontol A Biol Sci Med Sci* 2000;55:B286-B291.
24. Cha, YS and Sachan, DS. Oppostie effects of dietary saturated and unsaturated fatty acids on ethanol-pharmacokinetics, triglycerides and carnitines. *J Am Coll Nutr* 1994;13:338-343.
25. Ravnskov, U. The fallacies of the lipid hypothesis. *Scand Cardiovasc J* 2008;42:236-239.
26. Siri-Tarino, PW, et al. Meta-analysis of prospective cohort studies evaluating the association of saturated fat with cardiovascular disease. *American Journal of Clinical Nutrition* 2010;91:535-546.
27. Praagman, J, et al. The association between dietary saturated fatty acids and ischemic heart disease depends on the type and source of fatty acid in the European Prospective Investigation into Cancer and Nutrition-Netherlands cohort. *Am J Clin Nutr* 2016;103:356-365.
28. Grasgruber, P, et al. Food consumption and the actual statistics of cardiovascular diseases: an epidemiological comparison of 42 European countries. *Food Nutr Res* 2016;60:31694.
29. Dehghan, M, et al. Associations of fats and carbohydrate intake with cardio-vascular disease and mortality in 18 countries from five continents (PURE): a prospective cohort study. *Lancet* 2017;390:2050-2062.
30. Tewfik, IH, et al. The effect of intermittent heating on some chemical parame-ters of refined oils used in Egypt. A public health nutrition concern. *Int J Food Sci Nutr* 1998;49:339-342.
31. https://www.telegraph.co.uk/news/health/news/11981884/Cooking-with-vege-table-oils-releases-toxic-cancer-causing-chemicals-say-experts.html.
32. Raloff, J. 1996. Unusual fats lose heart-friendly image. *Science News* 1996;150:87.
33. Mensink, RP and Katan, MB. 1990. Effect of dietary trans fatty acids on high-density and low-density lipoprotein cholesterol levels in healthy subjects. *N Eng J Med* 323(7):439.
34. Willett, WC, et al. 1993. Intake of trans fatty acids and risk of coronary heart disease among women. *Lancet* 341(8845):581.
35. Booyens, J and Louwrens, CC. The Eskimo diet. Prophylactic effects ascribed to the balanced presence of natural cis unsaturated fatty acids and to the absence of unnatural trans and cis isomers of unsaturated fatty acids. *Med Hypoth* 1986;21:387.
36. Grandgirard, A., et al. Incorporation of trans long-chain n-3 polyunsaturated fatty acids in rat brain structures and retina. *Lipids* 1994;29:251-258.

Chapter 8: Fat Is A Superfood

1. Hung, MC, et al. Learning behavior and cerebral protein kinase C, antioxidant status, lipid composition in senescence-accelerated mouse: influence of a phosphatidylcholine-vitamin B12 diet. *British Journal of Nutrition* 2001;86:163-171.

2. Schneider, H, et al. Lipid based therapy for ulcerative colitis—modulation of intestinal mucus membrane phospholipids as a tool to influence inflammation. *Int J Mol Sci* 2010;11:4149-4164.

3. Kasbo, J, et al. Phosphatidyleholine-enriched diet prevents gallstone formation in mice susceptible to cholelithiasis. *Journal of Lipid Research* 2003;44:2297-2303.

4. Lim, YJ, et al. Advent of novel phosphatidylcholine-associated nonsteroidal anti-inflammatory drugs with improved gastrointestinal safety. *Gut Liver* 2013;7:7-15.

5. Kimura, I, et al. Short-chain fatty acids and ketones directly regulate sympathetic nervous system via G protein-coupled receptor 41 (GPR41). *PNAS* 2011;108:8030-8035.

6. Forsythe, CE, et al. Comparison of low fat and low carbohydrate diets on circulating fatty acid composition and markers for inflammation. *Lipids* 2008;43:65-77.

7. Kekwick, A. and Pawan, GLS. Calorie intake in relation to body weight changes in the obese. *Lancet* 1956;2:155.

8. Kekwick, A. and Pawan, G.L.S. Metabolic study in human obesity with isocaloric diets high in fat, protein or carbohydrate. *Metabolism* 1957;6:447-460.

9. Benoit, F, et al. Changes in body composition during weight reduction in obesity. *Archives of Internal Medicine*, 1965;63:604-612.

10. Vigilante, K. and Flynn, M. *Low-Fat Lies: High-Fat Frauds and the Healthiest Diet in the World*. Life Line Press: Washington, DC, 1999.

11. Goltz, SR, et al. Meal triacylglycerol profile modulates postprandial absorption of carotenoids in humans. *Mol Nutr Food Res* 2012;56:866-877.

12. Unlu, NZ, et al. Carotenoid absorption from salad and salsa by humans in enhanced by the addition of avocado or avocado oil. *J Nutr* 2005;135:431-436.

13. Vigilante, K and Flynn. *Low-Fat Lies: High-Fat Frauds and the Healthiest Diet in the World*. Life Line Press: Washington, DC, 1999.

14. Miura, S, et al. Modulation of intestinal immune system by dietary fat intake; relevance to Crohn's disease. *J Gastroenterol Hepatol* 1998;13:1183-1190.

15. Saketkhoo, K, et al. Effects of drinking hot water, cold water, and chicken soup on nasal mucus velocity and nasal airflow resistance. *Chest* 1978;74:408-410.

16. Hopkins, AB. Chicken soup cure may not be a myth. *Nurse Pract* 2003:28:16.

17. Rennard, BO, et al. Chicken soup inhibits neutrophil chemotaxis in vitro. *Chest* 2000;118:1150-1157.

18. Case Western Reserve University. "High fat diet reduces gut bacteria, Crohn's disease symptoms: Results could lead to new anti-inflammatory probiotics." *ScienceDaily*, 22 June 2017.

19. Khaw, KT, et al. Randomised trial of coconut oil, olive oil or butter on blood lipids and other cardiovascular risk factors in healthy men and women. *BMJ Open* 2018;8:e0290167.

20. Hayek, T, et al. Dietary fat increases high density lipoprotein (HDL) levels both by increasing the transport rates and decreasing the fractional catabolic rates of HDL cholesterol ester and apolipoprotein (Apo) A-I. Presentation of a new animal

model and mechanistic studies in human Apo A-I transgenic and control mice. *J Clin Invest* 1993;91:1665-1671.

21. Barbee, JF, et al. Apolipoproteins modulate the inflammatory response to lipopolysaccharide. *J Endotoxin* 2005:11:97-103.

22. Level, JH, et al. The protective effect of serum lipoproteins against bacterial lipopolysaccharide. *Eur Heart J* 1993;14:125-129.

23. Guo, L, et al. High density lipoprotein protects against polymicrobe-induced sepsis in mice. *J Biol Chem* 2013;288:17947-17953.

24. Iribarren, C, et al. Cohort study of serum total cholesterol and in-hospital incidence of infectious diseases. *Epidemiol Infect* 1998;121:335-347.

25. Ghoshal, S, et al. Chylomicrons promote intestinal absorption of lipopolysaccharides. *J Lipid Res* 2009;50:90-97.

26. Ravin, HA, et al. On the absorption of bacterial endotoxin from the gastro-intestinal tract of the normal and shocked animal. *J Exp Med* 1960;112:783-792.

27. Lyte, JM, et al. Postprandial serum endotoxin in healthy humans is modulated by dietary fat in a randomized, controlled, cross-over study. *Lipids Health Dis* 2016;15:186.

28. Nadhazi, Z, et al. Plasma endotoxin level of healthy donors. *Acta Microbial Immunol Hung* 2002;49:151-157.

29. Yang, H, et al. Energy metabolism in intestinal epithelial cells during maturation along the crypt-villus axis. *Scientific Reports* 2016;doi:10.1038/srep31917.

30. Hamer, H. M., et al. Review article: the role of butyrate on colonic function. *Aliment Pharmacol Ther* 200827:104-119.

31. Hu, G X, et al. Activation of the AMP activated protein kinase by short-chain fatty acids is the main mechanism underlying the beneficial effect of a high fiber diet on the metabolic syndrome. *Med Hypotheses* 2010;74: 123-126.

32. Gao, Z, et al. Butyrate improves insulin sensitivity and increases energy expenditure in mice. *Diabetes* 2009;58:1509-1517.

33. Blouin, J M, et al. Butyrate elicits a metabolic switch in human colon cancer cells by targeting the pyruvate dehydrogenase complex. *Int J Cancer* 2011;128: 2591-2601.

34. Harig, J M, et al. Treatment of diversion colitis with short-chain-fatty acid irrigation. *N Engl J Med* 1989;320: 23-28.

35. Di Sabatino, A, et al. Oral butyrate for mildly to moderately active Crohn's disease. *Alimen. Pharmacol Ther* 2005;22: 789-794.

36. Binder, H J. Role of colonic short-chain fatty acid transport in diarrhea. *Annu Rev Physiol* 2010:72: 297-313.

37. Jorgensen, JR, et al. In vivo absorption of medium-chain fatty acids by the rat colon exceeds that of short-chain fatty acids. *Gastroenterology* 2001;120:1152-1161.

38. Kono, H, et al. Dietary medium-chain triglycerides prevent chemically induced experimental colitis in rats. *Transl Res* 2010;155:131-141.

39. Kono, H, et al. Enteral diets enriched with medium-chain triglycerides and N-3 fatty acids prevent chemically induced experimental colitis in rats. *Transl Res* 2010;156:282-291.

40. Mane, J, et al. Partial replacement of dietary (n-6) fatty acids with medium-chain triglycerides decreases the incidence of spontaneous colitis in interleukin-10-deficient mice. *J Nutr* 2009;139:603-610.

41. Borrelli, O, et al. Polymeric diet alone versus corticosteroids in the treatment of active pediatric Crohn's disease: a randomized controlled open-label trial. *Clin Gastroenterol Hepatol* 2006;4:744-753.

42. Khoshoo, V, et al. Effect of low- and high-fat, peptide-based diets on body composition and disease activity in adolescents with active Crohn's disease. *JPEN J Parenter Enteral Nutr* 1996;20:401-405.

43. Tao, RC, et al. Glycerol: Its metabolism and use as an intravenous energy source. *Journal of Parenteral and Enteral Nutrition* 1983;7:479-488.

44. Tjonneland, A, et al. Linoleic acid, a dietary n-6 polyunsaturated fatty acid, and the aetiology of ulcerative colitis: a nested case-control study within a European prospective cohort study. *Gut* 2009;58(12):1606-1611.

45. Sarkar, A, et al. Psychobiotics and the manipulation of bacteria—gut brain signals. *Trends in Neurosciences* 2016;39:P763-781.

46. Turnbaugh, PJ, et al. An obesity-associated gut microbiome with increased capacity for energy harvest. *Nature* 2006;4444:1027-1031.

47. Bravo, JA, et al. Communication between gastrointestinal bacteria and the nervous system. *Curr Opin Pharmacol* 2012;12:667-672.

48. Lin, HV, et al. Butyrate and propionate protect against diet-induced obesity and regulate gut hormones via free fatty acid receptor 3-independent mechanisms. *PLoS ONE* 2012;7:e35240.

49. Pluznick, JL. Gut microbiota in renal physiology: focus on short-chain fatty acids and their receptors. *Kidney Int* 2016;90:119101198.

50. Nilsson, AG, et al. Lactobacillus reuteri reduces bone loss in older women with low bone mineral density—a randomized, placebo-controlled, double-blind, clinical trial. *Journal of Intern Med*; 2018. Doi:10.1111/joim.12805.

51. Sjogren, K., et al. The gut microbiota regulates bone mass in mice. *J Bone Miner Res* 2012;27:1357-1367.

52. Schott, EM, et al. Targeting the gut microbiome to treat the osteoarthritis of obesity. *JCI Insight* (2018). DOI: 10.1172/jci.insight.95997.

53. Dave Kolpack. Study shows high-fat diet might help pilots. Associated Press, October 7, 2009.

54. http://www.buffalo.edu/news/releases/1999/04/2793.html.

55. Volek, JS, et al. Rethinking fat as a fuel for endurance exercise. *Eur J Sport Sci* 2015;1:13-20.

56. Lambert, EV, et al. Nutritional strategies for promoting fat utilization and delaying the onset of fatigue during prolonged exercise. *J Sports Sci* 1997;15:315-324.

57. Phinney, SD, et al. Capacity for moderate exercise in obese subjects after adaptation to a hypocaloric ketogenic diet. *J Clin Invest* 1980;66:152-161.

58. Otto, M, et al. Serial measures of circulating biomarkers of dairy fat and total and cause-specific mortality in older adults: the Cardiovascular Health Study. *Am J Clin Nutr* 2018;108:476-484.

59. Gillman, MW, et al. Inverse association of dietary fat with dev elopement of ischemic stroke in men. *JAMA* 1997;278:2145-2150.

60. Monteiro, I and Vaz Almeid MD. Dietary fat and ischemic stroke risk in Northern Portugal. *Acta Med Port* 2007;20:307-318.

61. Mozaffarian, D, et al. Dietary fats, carbohydrate, and progression of coronary atherosclerosis in postmenopausal women. *Am J Clin Nutr* 2004;80:1175-1184.

62. Praagman, J, et al. The association between dietary saturated fatty acids and ischemic heart disease depends on the type and source of fatty acid in the European Prospective Investigation into Cancer and Nutrition-Netherlands cohort. *Am J Clin Nutr* 2016;103:356-365.

63. Grasgruber, P, et al. Food consumption and the actual statistics of cardiovascular diseases: an epidemiological comparison of 42 European countries. *Food Nutr Res* 2016;60:31694.

64. Dehghan, M, et al. Associations of fats and carbohydrate intake with cardiovascular disease and mortality in 18 countries form five continents (PURE): a prospective cohort study. *Lancet* 2017;390:2050-2062.

Chapter 9: Eat More Fat and Fewer Carbs

1. David Morgan, "Documentary: 'Fed Up' With Rising Childhood Obesity," CBS News, May 8, 2014, https://www.cbsnews.com/news/documentary-fed-up-with-rising-childhood-obesity/.

2. Cohen E, et al. Statistical review of US macronutrient consumption data, 1965–2011: Americans have been following dietary guidelines, coincident with the rise in obesity. *Nutrition* 2015;31:727–732.

3. Gross, LS, et al. Increased consumption of refined carbohydrates and the epidemic of type 2 diabetes in the United States: an ecological assessment. *Am J Clin Nutr* 2004;79:774-779.

4. Gardner, CD, et al. Comparison of the Atkins, Zone, Ornish, and LEARN diets for change in weight and related risk factors among overweight premenopausal women; the A to Z weight loss study: a randomized trial. *JAMA* 2007;297:969-977.

5. Forsythe, CE, et al. Comparison of low fat and low carbohydrate diets on circulating fatty acid composition and markers of inflammation. *Lipids* 2008;43:65-77.

6. Westman, EC, et al. The effect of a low-carbohydrate, ketogenic diet versus a low-glycemic index diet on glycemic control in type 2 diabetes mellitus. *Nutrition & Metabolism* 2008;5:36.

7. Yancy, WS, Jr, et al. A low-carbohydrate, ketogenic diet versus a low-fat diet to treat obesity and hyperlipidemia: a randomized, controlled trial. *Ann Intern Med* 2004;140:769-777.

8. Sharman, MJ, et al. Very low-carbohydrate and low-fat diets affect fasting lipids and postprandial lipemia differently in overweight men. *J Nutr* 2004;134:880-885.

9. Volek, JS, et al. Carbohydrate restriction has a more favorable impact on the metabolic syndrome than a low fat diet. *Lipids* 2009;44:297-309.

10. Tay, J, et al. Metabolic effects of weight loss on a very-low-carbohydrate diet compared with an isocaloric high-carbohydrate diet in abdominally obese subjects. *J Am Coll Card* 2008;51:59-67.

11. Keogh, JB, et al. Effects of weight loss from a very-low-carbohydrate diet on endothelial function and markers of cardiovascular disease risk in subjects with abdominal obesity. *Am J Clin Nutr* 2008;87:567-576.

12. Shai, I, et al. Weight loss with a low-carbohydrate, Mediterranean, or low-fat diet. *N Engl J Med* 2008;359:229-241.

13. Dyson, PA, et al. A low-carbohydrate diet is more effective in reducing body weight than healthy eating in both diabetic and non-diabetic subjects. *Diabetic Medicine* 2007;24:1430-1435.

14. McClernon, FJ, et al. The effects of a low-carbohydrate ketogenic diet and a low-fat diet on mood, hunger, and other self-reported symptoms. *Obesity (Silver Spring)* 2007;15:182-187.

15. Nickols-Richardson, SM, et al. Perceived hunger is lower and weight loss is greater in overweight premenopausal women consuming a low-carbohydrate/high-protein vs high-carbohydrate/low-fat diet. *J Am Dietetic Assoc* 2005;105:1433-1437.

Chapter 10: The Ketogenic Diet

1. Reger, MA, et al. Effects of beta-hydroxybutyrate on cognition in memory-impaired adults. *Neurobiol Aging* 2004;25:311-314.

2. Kashiwaya, Y, et al. D-beta-hydroxybutyrate protects neurons in models of Alzheimer's and Parkinson's disease. *Proc Natl Acad Sci USA* 2000;97:5440-5444..

3. VanItallie, TB, et al. Treatment of Parkinson disease with diet-induced hyperketonemia: a feasibility study. *Neurology* 2005;64:728-730.

4. Zhao, W, et al. Caprylic triglyceride as a novel therapeutic approach to effectively improve the performance and attenuate the symptoms due to the motor neuron loss in ALS disease. *PLoS One* 2012;7(11):e49191.

5. Appleberg, S, et al. Ketogenic diet improves recovery of function after traumatic brain injury in juvenile rats. *J Neurotrama* 2007;24:1267.

6. Prins, ML. Cerebral metabolic adaptation and ketone metabolism after brain injury. *J Cereb Blood Flow Metab* 2008;28:1-16.

7. Maggioni, F, et al. Ketogenic diet in migraine treatment: a brief but ancient history. *Cephalalgia* 2011;31:1150-1151.

8. Kossoff, EH, et al. Use of the modified Atkins diet for adolescents with chronic daily headache. *Cephalalgia* 2010;30:1014-1016.

9. Husain, AM, et al. Diet therapy for narcolepsy. *Neurology* 2004;62:2300-2302.

10. Kim, DY, et al. Inflammation-mediated memory dysfunction and effects of a ketogenic diet in a murine model of multiple sclerosis. *PLoS One* 1012;7:e35476.

11. Murphy, P, et al. The antidepressant properties of the ketogenic diet. *Biol Psychiatry* 2004;56:981-983.

12. Nebeling, LC, et al. Effects of a ketogenic diet on tumor metabolism and nutritional status in pediatric oncology patients: two case reports. *J Am Coll Nutr* 1995;14:202-208.

13. Sharman, MJ, et al. Very low-carbohydrate and low-fat diets affect fasting lipids and postprandial lipemia differently in overweight men. *J Nutr* 2004;134:880-885.

14. Yancy, WS, Jr, et al. A low-carbohydrate, ketogenic diet versus a low-fat diet to treat obesity and hyperlipidemia: a randomized, controlled trial. *Ann Intern Med* 2004;140:769-777.

15. Westman, EC, et al. Low-carbohydrate nutrition and metabolism. *Am J Clin Nutr* 2007;86:276-284.

16. Westman, EC, et al. A review of low-carbohydrate ketogenic diets. *Curr Atheroscler Rep* 2003;5:476-483.

17. Westman, EC, et al. The effect of a low-carbohydrate, ketogenic diet versus a low-glycemic index diet on glycemic control in type 2 diabetes mellitus. *Nutr Metab (Lond)* 2008;5:36.

18. Sharman, MJ, et al. Very low-carbohydrate and low-fat diets affect fasting lipids and postprandial lipemia differently in overweight men. *J Nutr* 2004;134:880-885.

19. Gardner, CD, et al. Comparison of the Atkins, Zone, Ornish, and LEARN diets for change in weight and related risk factors among overweight premenopausal women: The A to Z Weight Loss Study: A randomized trial. *JAMA* 2007;297:969-977.

20. Volek, JS and Sharman, MJ. Cardiovascular and hormonal aspects of very-low-carbohydrate ketogenic diets. *Obes Res* 2004;12 Suppl 2:115S-123S.

21. Sherman, MJ, et al A ketogenic diet favorably affects serum biomarkers for cardiovascular disease in normal-weight men. *J Nutr* 2002;132:1879-1885.

22. Foster, GD, et al. Weight and metabolic outcomes after 2 years on a low-carbohydrate versus low-fat diet: A randomized trial. *Ann Intern Med* 2010;153:147-157.

23. Maalouf, M, et al. Ketones inhibit mitochondrial production of reactive oxygen species production following glutamate excitotoxicity by increasing NADH oxidation. *Neuroscience* 2007;145:256-264.

24. Stafford, P, et al. The ketogenic diet reverses gene expression patterns and reduces reactive oxygen species levels when used as an adjuvant therapy for glioma. *Nutrition & Metabolism* 2010;7:74.

25. Shimazu, T, et al. Suppression of oxidative stress by beta-hydroxybutyrate, an endogenous histone deacetylase inhibitor. *Science* 2013;339:211-214.

26. Veech, RL. The therapeutic implications of ketone bodies: the effects of ketone bodies in pathological conditions: ketosis, ketogenic diet, redox states, insulin resistance, and mitochondrial metabolism. *Prostaglandins Leukot Essent Fatty Acids* 2004;70:309-319.

27. Kashiwaya, Y, et al. A ketone ester diet increased brain malonyl CoA and uncoupling protein 4 and 5 while decreasing food intake in the normal Wistar rat. *J Biol Chem* 2010;285:25950-25956.

28. Kashiwaya, Y, et al. Substrte signaling by insulin: a ketone bodies ratio mimics insulin action in heart. *Am J Cardiol* 1997;80:50A-64A.

29. Youm, YH, et al. The ketone metabolite beta-hydroxybutyrate blocks NLRP3 inflammasome-mediated inflammatory disease. *Nat Med* 2015;21:263-266.

30. Veech, RL. The therapeutic implications of ketone bodies: the effects of ketone bodies in pathologic conditions: ketosis, ketogenic diet, redox states, insulin resistance, and mitochondrial metabolism. *Prostaglandins Leukol Essent Fatty Acids* 2004;70:309-319.

31. Hasselbalch, SG, et al. Changes in cerebral blood flow and carbohydrate metabolism during acute hyperketonemia. *Am J Physiol* 1996;270:E746-751.

32. Marie, C, et al. Fasting prior to transient cerebral ischemia reduces delayed neuronal necrosis. *Metab Bran Dis* 1990;5:65-75.

33. Prins, ML, et al. Increased cerebral uptake and oxidation of exogenous βHB improves ATP following traumatic brain injury in adult rats. *J Neurochem* 2004;90:666-672.

34. Suzuki, M, et al. Effect of β-hydroxybutyrate, a cerebral function improving agent, on cerebral hypoxia, anoxia and ischemia in mice and rats. *Jpn J Pharmacol* 2001;87:143-150.

35. Maalouf, M, et al. The neuroprotective properties of calorie restriction, the ketogenic diet, and ketone bodies. *Brain Res Rev* 2009; 59:293-315.

36. Koper, JW, et al. Acetoacetate and glucose as substrates for lipid synthesis for rat brain oligodendrocytes and astrocytes in serum-free culture. *Biochim Biophys Acta* 1984;796:20-26.

37. Kashiwaya, Y, et al. A ketone ester diet exhibits anxiolytic and cognition-sparing properties, and lessens amyloid and tau pathologies in a mouse model of Alzheimer's disease. *Neurobiol Aging* 2013;34:1530-1539.

38. Hemderson, ST. Ketone bodies as a therapeutic for Alzheimer's disease. *Neurotherapeutics* 2008;5:470-480.

39. Henderson ST, et al. Study of the ketogenic agent AC-1202 in mild to moderate Alzheimer's disease: a randomized, double-blind, placebo-controlled, multicenter trial. *Nutr Metab (London)* 2009; 6:31.doi:10.1186/1743-7075-6-31.

40. Veech, RL. Ketone ester effects on metabolism and transcription. *J Lipid Res* 2014;55:2004-2006.

41. Poff, AM, et al. Ketone supplementation decreases tumor cell viability and prolongs survival of mice with metastatic cancer. *Int J Cancer* 22014;135:1711-1720.

42. Shukla, SK, et al. Metabolic reprogramming induced by ketone bodies diminishes pancreatic cancer cachexia. *Cancer Metab* 2014;2:18.

43. Rossi, AP, et al. Abstract 3346; the ketone body beta-hydroxybutyrate increases radiosensitivity in giloma cell lines in vitro. *Cancer Res* 2015;75:3346. doi: 10.1158/1538-7445.am2015-3346.

44. Scheck, AC, et al. The ketogenic diet for the treatment of glioma: insights from genetic profiling. *Epilepsy Res* 2012;100:327-337.

45. Newman, JC and Verdin, E. Ketone bodies as signaling metabolites. *Trends Endocrinol Metab* 2014;25;42-52.

46. Stafford, P, et al. The ketogenic diet reverses gene expression patterns and reduces reactive oxygen species levels when used as an adjuvant therapy for glioma. *Nutr Metab (London)* 2010;7:74. doi: 10.1186/1743-7075-7-74.

47. Siddalingaswamy, M, et al. Anti-diabetic effects of cold and heat extracted virgin coconut oil. *JDM* 2011;1:118-123.

48. Fife, B. *The Stevia Deception: The Hidden Dangers of Low-Calorie Sweeteners.* Piccadilly Books, Ltd.: Colorado Springs, CO, 2017.

49. Volek, JS, et al. Rethinking fat as a fuel for endurance exercise. *European J Sport Sci* 2015;15:13-20.

50. http://www.gpo.gov/fdsys/pkg/FR-1995-07-20/pdf/95-17505.pdf.

51. Johnson, RK, et al. Dietary sugars intake and cardiovascular health: A scientific statement from the American Heart Association. *Circulation* 2009;120:1011-1020.

Index

Ketone Therapy
The Ketogenic Cleanse and Anti-Aging Diet

The ketogenic diet is one that is very low in carbohydrate, high in fat, with moderate protein. This diet shifts the body into a natural, healthy metabolic state known as nutritional ketosis.

Low-fat diets have been heavily promoted for the past several decades as the answer to obesity and chronic disease. However, we are fatter and sicker now more than ever before. Obviously, the low-fat approach has not worked. Our bodies actually need fat for optimal health and function more efficiently using fat for fuel.

In this book you will discover how people are successfully using ketones and the ketogenic diet to prevent and treat chronic and degenerative disease. Topics covered include, weight loss; neurodegenerative disorders such as Alzheimer's and Parkinson's disease; neurodevelopmental disorders, such as ADHD and autism; diabetes and metabolic syndrome; eyesight; detoxification and immune function; digestive health; cancer, and more.

Ketone therapy is backed by decades of medical and clinical research, which has proven the method to be both safe and effective for the treatment of variety of health issues,.

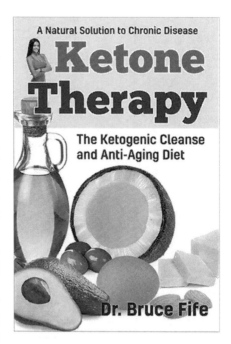

Many health problems that medical science has deemed incurable or untreatable are being reversed. Medications that were once relied on daily are no longer necessary and are being tossed away. People are discovering that a simple, but revolutionary diet based on wholesome, natural foods and the most health-promoting fats is dramatically changing their lives.

This book describes the ketogenic diet in detail and how to incorporate it into your life to prevent and overcome chronic disease.

Low-Carb, High-Fat Bookshelf

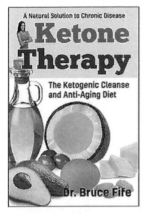
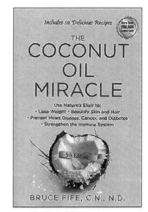
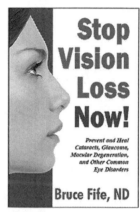

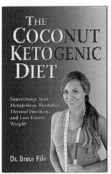
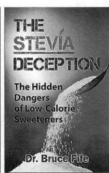
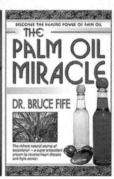
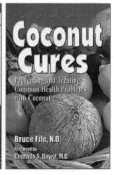

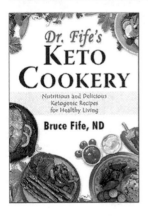
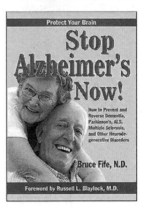
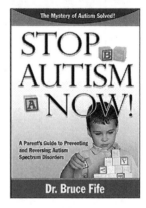

Visit Us on the Web

PB Piccadilly Books, Ltd.

www.piccadillybooks.com

Made in the USA
Lexington, KY
20 March 2019